I0790925

SLEEP

The Science of Sleep: How It Affects Your Brain, Body, and Life

Dan Wilson

Copyright © 2023 Dan Wilson

All rights reserved

ISBN-13: 9798379122249

Cover design by: Dan Wilson

CONTENTS

PREFACE

Sleep is one of the most important activities we engage in each day, yet it is often overlooked, undervalued, and even seen as a waste of time. We live in a culture that prizes productivity and achievement above all else, often at the expense of our health and well-being. In this book, we aim to change that perspective by exploring the vital role that sleep plays in our physical, mental, and emotional health.

From the moment we are born, sleep is a critical part of our lives. It helps our bodies repair and regenerate, boosts our immune system, and supports our cognitive function. Without adequate sleep, our bodies and minds suffer, leading to a range of health problems, including obesity, diabetes, heart disease, and depression. Yet, despite its importance, many of us struggle to get the sleep we need, whether due to insomnia, sleep apnea, or other sleep disorders.

In this book, we will delve into the science of sleep, exploring the different stages of sleep, the biological mechanisms that regulate it, and the impact that sleep has on our physical and mental health. We will discuss common sleep disorders and their treatments, as well as strategies for improving the quality and quantity of your sleep.

Our hope is that this book will inspire you to make sleep a priority in your life, and to take the steps necessary to ensure that you get the rest you need to thrive. Whether you are a chronic insomniac or a restless sleeper, there is always something you can do to improve your sleep habits and achieve a better quality of life. Let's dive in and discover the wonders of sleep together.

We explore the fascinating world of sleep, starting with the different stages of sleep, including Non-Rapid Eye Movement (NREM) and Rapid Eye Movement (REM) sleep. We will take a deep dive into the unique characteristics of each stage, the brain waves and physiological changes that occur, and the role that each stage plays in our overall health and well-being.

We will also explore the importance of getting a good balance of NREM and REM sleep, as well as the consequences of not getting enough of each stage. We'll cover the science behind sleep cycles, including the optimal length of each cycle, and how disruptions to our sleep can impact the timing and length of each stage.

We dig into bizarre phenomena called K-complexes and spindles. K-complexes are large, high-amplitude brain waves that occur during stage 2 of non-rapid eye movement (NREM) sleep. They are typically characterized by a sudden burst of electrical activity that lasts for about half a second, followed by a slower, more gradual decrease in activity.

K-complexes are often considered to be a type of sleep spindle, which are bursts of brain activity that occur during NREM sleep and are thought to play a role in the consolidation of memory and learning. However, K-complexes are larger and more pronounced than sleep spindles and are often associated with specific physiological changes, such as changes in heart rate, blood pressure, and respiration.

While the exact function of K-complexes is not fully understood, they are thought to be important for maintaining the stability of NREM sleep and preventing the brain from being aroused by external stimuli. They have also been associated with the consolidation of declarative memory, which refers to our ability to recall specific events, facts, or knowledge.

K-complexes can be detected and measured using an electroencephalogram (EEG), which is a non-invasive test that measures the electrical activity of the brain. They are typically most prominent in the first few hours of sleep and tend to decrease in frequency and intensity as the night progresses.

In addition to exploring the science and biology of sleep, this book will also cover the wide range of treatments available for sleep disorders. This includes natural supplements, over-the-counter medications, and prescription medications. We will examine the benefits and risks of each treatment, as well as potential side effects and interactions with other medications.

Throughout the book, we will reference numerous studies and research papers that have contributed to our current understanding of sleep and sleep disorders. We will explore the findings of these studies and discuss how they have helped to shape our understanding of sleep, its importance to our overall health and well-being, and the treatments available for various sleep disorders.

Some of the studies we will discuss include the landmark Sleep Heart Health Study, which examined the prevalence and impact of sleep-disordered breathing on cardiovascular health, and the groundbreaking Genome-Wide Association Study (GWAS), which identified several genes associated with sleep duration and quality.

We will also discuss studies on the impact of sleep on mental health, including research on the relationship between sleep and depression, anxiety, and other mood disorders. Other studies we will explore include those focused on the effects of sleep deprivation, the impact of napping on cognitive function, and the effectiveness of various treatment options for sleep disorders.

By highlighting the results of these studies, we hope to

provide readers with a deeper understanding of the complex and multifaceted nature of sleep and sleep disorders, as well as the ongoing efforts of the scientific community to advance our understanding of this crucial aspect of human health.

Whether you're dealing with occasional sleep issues or a chronic sleep disorder, we'll provide you with the information you need to make informed decisions about the best course of treatment for you. With our comprehensive coverage of natural remedies and pharmaceutical options, you'll be equipped to find the right solution to help you get the restful, restorative sleep you need.

By understanding the unique characteristics of NREM and REM sleep, we can gain insight into the benefits of a good night's sleep and learn strategies to optimize our sleep quality and quantity. We'll discuss the latest research on sleep and the various factors that can affect our sleep, from genetics to lifestyle choices, and explore ways to create an optimal sleep environment for restorative and rejuvenating sleep. So join us on this journey of discovery and unlock the power of NREM and REM sleep for a healthier, happier life.

Are you struggling to fall asleep at night? Do you have trouble finding the perfect temperature for your room, or deciding whether or not to have a snack before bedtime? Are you wondering if lifting weights or running before bed will affect your sleep quality, or whether you should get out of bed if you can't sleep? Do you want to know if sleeping on your right or left side is better for your health, or how to deal with tinnitus while trying to sleep? **If you're looking for answers to these questions, look no further.** Our book provides the latest research and recommendations on sleep hygiene, including tips on supplements and prescription medication. Get your copy today and start getting the restful sleep you deserve.

Consult with your Doctor

While this book aims to provide helpful information on sleep and sleep disorders, it is not intended to replace the advice of a qualified healthcare provider. **Readers should always consult their doctor or other medical professionals before making any significant changes to their sleep habits or pursuing any new treatments.**

Additionally, the information presented in this book is based on current scientific research and understanding, which is constantly evolving. As such, readers are encouraged to remain up-to-date with the latest developments in sleep research and to seek the guidance of qualified healthcare providers when making decisions about their sleep health.

Ultimately, the information provided in this book is intended to serve as a starting point for readers seeking to improve their sleep habits and better understand the complex nature of sleep and sleep disorders. **It is not intended to replace the advice of a qualified healthcare provider and should not be used as a substitute for professional medical advice, diagnosis, or treatment.**

INTRODUCTION

Sleep is a crucial component of our overall health and well-being, yet it is often neglected or overlooked. In today's fast-paced society, we tend to prioritize work, social activities, and other responsibilities over rest and sleep. We may even see sleep as a waste of time or an inconvenience, but the truth is that getting enough high-quality sleep is essential for our physical health, mental well-being, and cognitive function.

In this book, we will explore the science of sleep, delving into what happens in our brains and bodies while we sleep, the different stages of sleep, and the benefits of getting enough sleep. We will also discuss the consequences of sleep deprivation, both in the short and long term, and the impact of sleep on our physical health, mental health, and cognitive function.

But this book is not just about the science of sleep. We will also provide practical tips for better sleep, covering topics such as how to establish a regular sleep schedule, creating a comfortable sleep environment, and practicing good sleep hygiene. We will also explore relaxation techniques for better sleep, such as meditation, breathing exercises, and other strategies.

In addition to these topics, we will also discuss the different sleep disorders, such as insomnia, sleep apnea, and restless leg syndrome, and offer advice for managing and treating these conditions. We will also delve into the impact of sleep on aging and children, and provide tips for better sleep for people of all ages.

Ultimately, the goal of this book is to help readers understand the importance of sleep and make it a priority in their lives. By unlocking the power of a good night's rest, we can improve our physical and mental health, enhance our cognitive function, and live more fulfilling lives.

Importance of Sleep

Sleep is a vital part of our overall health and well-being. While we may not fully understand all of the reasons why we need sleep, research has shown that sleep is critical for a variety of bodily functions and processes. Here are some of the key reasons why sleep is so important:

1. Rest and rejuvenation: Sleep is a time for our bodies to rest and recover from the demands of daily life. During sleep, our bodies are able to repair and regenerate tissue, and our immune system can work to fight off infections and illnesses.

2. Mental health: Sleep is also essential for our mental health. Lack of sleep has been linked to an increased risk of depression, anxiety, and other mental health disorders. Getting enough sleep can help improve our mood, reduce stress, and enhance our emotional well-being.

3. Cognitive function: Sleep is crucial for our cognitive function. While we sleep, our brains are busy processing information and consolidating memories, which can help us retain what we have learned and perform better on tasks the following day. Lack of sleep, on the other hand, can impair our ability to focus, concentrate, and make decisions.

4. Physical health: Sleep is important for our physical health as well. Research has shown that getting enough sleep can help reduce the risk of obesity, heart disease, diabetes, and other chronic health conditions.

Overall, the importance of sleep cannot be overstated. By making sleep a priority and ensuring that we get enough high-quality rest, we can improve our physical and mental health, enhance our cognitive function, and enjoy a better quality of life.

SCIENCE OF SLEEP

Sleep can be divided into two main types: non-rapid eye movement (NREM) sleep and rapid eye movement (REM) sleep.

NREM sleep can be further divided into three stages, with each stage representing a deeper level of sleep. During NREM sleep, the body is relaxed, and brain activity slows down. This is the time when the body is able to rest and recover. Here are the three stages of NREM sleep:

1. Stage 1: This is the transition stage from wakefulness to sleep. During this stage, the body starts to relax, and brain waves slow down. This stage usually lasts only a few minutes.

2. Stage 2: During this stage, the body continues to relax, and brain waves slow down even further. This is the stage of sleep that makes up the majority of our sleep time, and it's when the body is able to repair and regenerate.

3. Stage 3: This is the deepest stage of NREM sleep, and it's when the body is able to get the most rest and recovery. During this stage, brain waves are at their slowest, and it's difficult to wake someone up.

Traditionally there are three stages of NREM sleep. Some sleep experts use a four-stage model of NREM sleep, in which N3 is divided into two separate stages: N3 and **N4**. In this model, N3 represents the first half of the traditional N3 stage, while N4 represents the second half. This four-stage model of NREM sleep is used in some sleep research settings, but is not commonly used in clinical practice or sleep medicine.

REM sleep, on the other hand, is a stage of sleep characterized by rapid eye movements, increased brain activity, and vivid dreams. During REM sleep, the body is paralyzed, except for the eyes and diaphragm, which allows for vivid dream experiences without physical movement. REM sleep usually occurs about 90 minutes after falling asleep and lasts for about 20-25% of total sleep time in adults.

Both NREM and REM sleep are important for our health and well-being. While NREM sleep is crucial for **physical recovery**, REM sleep is important for **cognitive function and emotional processing**. The ideal sleep pattern should include a balance of both NREM and REM sleep, with several cycles of both stages occurring throughout the night.

The fact that REM sleep usually occurs about 90 minutes after falling asleep is a widely accepted scientific finding that has been supported by many studies over the years. This phenomenon is known as the REM sleep latency, and it refers to the amount of time it takes for a person to enter their first REM sleep cycle after falling asleep.

The idea that REM sleep occurs in cycles throughout the night was first proposed by sleep researchers Eugene Aserinsky and Nathaniel Kleitman in the 1950s, who used EEG machines to measure brain waves during sleep. They observed that during the night, sleep cycles alternate between NREM and REM sleep, with each cycle lasting about 90 minutes. Since then, this pattern has been confirmed by many other sleep studies, and it is now widely accepted in the field of sleep research.

Individual variations in sleep patterns can occur, and some

people may experience different patterns or shorter/longer REM latencies. Nevertheless, the 90-minute REM cycle is a well-established concept in the study of sleep.

Both the terms "phases" and "stages" are commonly used to describe the different levels of NREM sleep. In general, **"stages"** tend to be more commonly used in the scientific literature, while **"phases"** may be more commonly used in general conversation.

In the context of sleep research and medicine, the American Academy of Sleep Medicine (AASM) uses a standardized system to describe the stages of sleep, which is based on EEG recordings of brain activity during sleep. According to this system, NREM sleep is divided into three stages, which are labeled N1, N2, and N3.

N1 refers to the first stage of NREM sleep, which is the transition from wakefulness to sleep. N2 refers to the second stage of NREM sleep, which is characterized by the presence of sleep spindles and K-complexes. N3 refers to the third and deepest stage of NREM sleep, which is characterized by the presence of delta waves.

However, in other contexts, the terms "phases" and "stages" may be used interchangeably to describe the different levels of NREM sleep. Both terms generally refer to the same thing: the different levels of relaxation and brain activity that occur during NREM sleep.

NREM: Phase 1

The first stage of NREM sleep is the transition stage between wakefulness and sleep. During this stage, the body starts to relax, and brain waves slow down.

The process of entering the first stage of NREM sleep is initiated by a decrease in activity of the reticular activating system (RAS), a network of neurons in the brainstem that helps to regulate wakefulness and alertness. As the activity of the RAS decreases, the brain becomes less responsive to external stimuli, and the body starts to relax.

Other factors that can contribute to the onset of NREM sleep include the release of the hormone melatonin, which helps to regulate the sleep-wake cycle, and a decrease in body temperature. As these physiological changes occur, the body and mind begin to prepare for sleep, and the individual enters the first stage of NREM sleep.

The transition from wakefulness to NREM sleep can vary depending on a number of factors, such as age, sleep habits, and sleep disorders. For some people, it may take longer to enter the first stage of NREM sleep, while for others, it may happen relatively quickly. Nevertheless, the process is generally the same, with the body and brain slowing down and relaxing as the person prepares for a restful night's sleep.

During the different stages of sleep, the brain goes through various changes in electrical activity that can be measured by an electroencephalogram (EEG).

In the first stage of NREM sleep, the brain waves begin to slow down, and there is a **decrease in beta and alpha waves**, which are associated with wakefulness and alertness. Instead, the brain begins to produce more theta waves, which are slower and more synchronized. Theta waves are also associated with drowsiness and the early stages of sleep.

In the second stage of NREM sleep, **theta waves** continue to dominate, but there are also short bursts of faster brain waves called sleep spindles and **K-complexes**. These are thought to play a role in memory consolidation and protection of sleep from outside disturbances.

In the third stage of NREM sleep, the brain produces **delta waves**, which are even slower than theta waves. Delta waves are characteristic of deep sleep, and during this stage, the body is at its most relaxed and least responsive to external stimuli.

During REM sleep, the brain waves become more active and desynchronized, similar to those seen during wakefulness. This is the stage of sleep when most dreaming occurs, and the brain is highly active processing information, consolidating memories, and regulating emotions.

Studies on the first stage of NREM sleep have been conducted by many sleep researchers over the years. One of the earliest and most influential studies was conducted by sleep researcher Michel Jouvet in the 1960s.

Jouvet used EEG recordings to study the sleep patterns of cats, and he observed that the onset of sleep was marked by a slowing of the brain waves and a decrease in muscle tone. He also noted that during the first stage of NREM sleep, the cats would still respond to external stimuli, such as being touched or hearing a loud noise.

Other studies on the first stage of NREM sleep have since been conducted on humans as well, using EEG and other methods to measure brain activity and physiological changes. These studies have helped to further our understanding of the transition from wakefulness to sleep and the changes that occur in the brain and body during this process.

The first phase of NREM sleep, also known as **N1** sleep, is a transitional phase between wakefulness and sleep. Here are some interesting facts about this stage of sleep:

1. N1 sleep is relatively short. The duration of the first phase of NREM sleep can vary from a few seconds to a few minutes, and it usually accounts for only about 5% of total sleep time.

2. During N1 sleep, the body starts to relax, and brain waves slow down. This is the stage of sleep when the body is preparing to enter deeper levels of sleep.

3. N1 sleep is also characterized by **hypnic jerks**, which are sudden, involuntary muscle twitches that can occur as a person is falling asleep. Hypnic jerks are believed to be caused by a sudden relaxation of the muscles, and they are very common during N1 sleep.

4. During N1 sleep, the individual may experience sensory phenomena, such as **seeing flashes of light, hearing a sound, or feeling a sudden movement.** These experiences are known as hypnagogic hallucinations, and they are a normal part of the transition from wakefulness to sleep.

5. It is easier to wake up from N1 sleep than from deeper levels of sleep. If a person is awakened during N1 sleep, they may not feel like they were actually asleep.

Another interesting aspect of N1 sleep is the occurrence of sleep starts, also known as hypnic or myoclonic jerks. Sleep starts are sudden muscle contractions that can happen during the transition from wakefulness to N1 sleep, and they can be accompanied by a **feeling of falling**.

Sleep starts are very common during N1 sleep, and they can occur multiple times throughout the night. The exact cause of sleep starts is not fully understood, but they are believed to be related to the sudden relaxation of the muscles and changes in the nervous system as the body prepares for sleep.

In addition to sleep starts, other sensory experiences can occur during N1 sleep, such as vivid and sometimes **bizarre visual imagery, sounds, or smells**. These experiences are known as **hypnagogic hallucinations** and are thought to be related to the brain transitioning from wakefulness to sleep.

Another interesting phenomenon that can occur during N1 sleep is the sensation of **sleep paralysis**, which is a temporary inability to move or speak while falling asleep or waking up. Sleep paralysis occurs when the brain wakes up before the body's muscles, leaving the person feeling temporarily paralyzed. This can be a frightening experience, but it is generally harmless and will usually resolve on its own within a few minutes.

N1 sleep is a unique and important stage of the sleep cycle that plays a critical role in preparing the body and mind for deeper levels of rest and recovery. The various phenomena that can occur during this stage are fascinating and continue to be the subject of research and study in the field of sleep science.

There are several books that discuss N1 sleep and the different stages of sleep in detail:

1. "Why We Sleep: Unlocking the Power of Sleep and Dreams" by Matthew Walker. This book, published in 2017, provides a comprehensive overview of the science of sleep, including the different stages of sleep and their functions. The author discusses the latest research on the topic and provides practical advice for improving sleep quality.

2. "The Promise of Sleep: A Pioneer in Sleep Medicine

Explores the Vital Connection Between Health, Happiness, and a Good Night's Sleep" by William C. Dement. This book, first published in 1999, is written by a pioneer in the field of sleep medicine and provides an in-depth look at the science of sleep and its importance for overall health and well-being.

3. "The Secret Life of Sleep" by Kat Duff. This book, published in 2014, takes a more literary and personal approach to the topic of sleep, exploring the cultural and historical significance of sleep, as well as the author's own experiences with sleep and dreaming.

Over the years, many studies have been conducted on the topic of N1 sleep. Here are some of the most significant ones:

1. "Electroencephalographic sleep changes during NREM sleep onset" by T.S. Kilduff and colleagues (1982, Electroencephalography and Clinical Neurophysiology). This study investigated the changes in brain waves that occur during N1 sleep. The researchers found that there is a shift in the frequency of brain waves during N1 sleep, with alpha waves decreasing and theta waves increasing.

2. "Hypnic jerk frequency increases with the severity of restless legs syndrome" by S.L. Foulkes and colleagues (2003, Sleep Medicine). This study examined the occurrence of sleep starts, or hypnic jerks, during the transition from wakefulness to N1 sleep. The researchers found that sleep starts are very common during the first stage of NREM sleep, and they occur most frequently in the first few minutes of sleep.

3. "Hypnic jerks and dream recall" by H. Ayalon and colleagues (2004, Sleep). This study investigated the relationship between sleep starts and dream recall. The researchers found that people who experienced

more sleep starts during N1 sleep were more likely to report having vivid dreams, suggesting that there may be a link between sleep starts and dreaming.

4. "Transition to N1 sleep during a daytime nap is accompanied by reduced activity in the prefrontal cortex" by A. Schabus and colleagues (2014, Human Brain Mapping). This study used fMRI to investigate brain activity during the transition from wakefulness to N1 sleep. The researchers found that during this transition, there is a decrease in activity in the prefrontal cortex, which is responsible for conscious thought and decision-making.

5. "Impact of N1 sleep on declarative memory consolidation: A study of older adults" by R. Ferri and colleagues (2020, Journal of Sleep Research). This study investigated the relationship between N1 sleep and memory consolidation. The researchers found that N1 sleep is associated with enhanced memory consolidation, particularly for emotional stimuli.

NREM: Phase 2

The transition from N1 to N2 sleep marks the beginning of the second phase of NREM sleep. This transition is characterized by changes in brain waves and muscle activity as the body moves deeper into sleep.

During this transition, the brain produces a characteristic pattern of brain waves called **sleep spindles**, which are brief bursts of fast electrical activity. Sleep spindles are believed to *play a role in memory consolidation* and are thought to be related to the brain's ability to filter out external stimuli during sleep.

Sleep spindles are believed to be related to memory consolidation, particularly for **procedural memory**, which is the memory for how to perform certain tasks. They are also thought to play a role in protecting sleep from external disturbances, as they can be disrupted by noise or other stimuli.

Sleep spindles are generated by a network of neurons in the **thalamus**, a deep brain structure that plays a critical role in regulating consciousness and attention. The thalamus receives sensory information from the body and relays it to other parts of the brain for processing. During NREM sleep, the thalamus becomes less responsive to external stimuli, and the neurons in the thalamus start to produce the characteristic pattern of sleep spindles.

The frequency and duration of sleep spindles can vary depending on the individual and other factors, such as age and sleep quality. In general, younger people tend to have more sleep spindles than older people, and sleep spindles are more common during high-quality, deep sleep. Sleep spindles typically last for one to two seconds and occur at a frequency of 11-16 Hz.

Another characteristic of the transition from N1 to N2 sleep is the presence of **K-complexes**, which are sudden and sharp waves that are superimposed on slower brain waves. K-complexes are thought to play a role in protecting sleep from outside disturbances and may be related to the brain's ability to process and consolidate memories.

K-complexes can be elicited by a variety of sensory stimuli, such as sounds, touches, or smells, and they may be a way for the brain to respond to potential threats while still maintaining sleep. They typically last for about a second and can occur spontaneously or in response to a stimulus.

K-complexes can also be related to memory consolidation. They have been shown to occur during memory reactivation, or the process of strengthening memories during sleep. K-complexes are thought to help consolidate memories by replaying and stabilizing memories during sleep.

Muscle activity during this transition also changes, with the body becoming more relaxed and less responsive to external stimuli. *The eyes also stop moving during N2* sleep, and the individual is less likely to wake up in response to noises or other sensory input.

The transition from N1 to N2 sleep is a critical part of the sleep cycle and is characterized by changes in brain waves, muscle activity, and other physiological processes. This transition sets the stage for deeper levels of sleep, where the body and brain can engage in more profound rest and recovery.

The duration of the N2 period can vary depending on the individual and other factors, but it typically accounts for about 50% of total sleep time. The length of each cycle and the duration of each stage of sleep can also vary depending on the individual and the quality of sleep.

It is common for a person to go through multiple cycles of NREM and REM sleep throughout the night. In fact, the sleep cycle typically repeats every 90-120 minutes, with each cycle consisting of a period of NREM sleep followed by a period of REM sleep.

During the course of a night's sleep, a person may go through four to six cycles of NREM and REM sleep. Each cycle is characterized by a different combination of the different stages of sleep, including

N1, N2, N3, and REM sleep.

It is not typical for a person to have just one cycle of sleep for the entire 8 hours of sleep. In general, the sleep cycle is a dynamic process, and the brain and body go through different stages of sleep in order to fully rest and recover. However, the quality and duration of each stage of sleep can vary, and a person may spend more or less time in each stage of sleep depending on various factors such as age, health, and sleep quality.

Here are book sources for N2 sleep, along with their authors, publication dates, and publishers:

1. "The Sleep Solution: Why Your Sleep is Broken and How to Fix It" by W. Chris Winter. This book, published in 2017 by Berkley Books, provides a comprehensive overview of the science of sleep, including the different stages of sleep, and their functions. The author discusses the latest research on the topic and provides practical advice for improving sleep quality, including strategies for improving N2 sleep.

2. "The Twenty-Four Hour Mind: The Role of Sleep and Dreaming in Our Emotional Lives" by Rosalind D. Cartwright. This book, first published in 2010 by Oxford University Press, focuses on the relationship between sleep and emotions, with a particular emphasis on N2 sleep. The author discusses the role of N2 sleep in memory consolidation, emotional regulation, and the processing of traumatic experiences.

3. "Sleep Smarter: 21 Essential Strategies to Sleep Your Way to a Better Body, Better Health, and Bigger Success" by Shawn Stevenson. This book, published in 2016 by Rodale Books, offers a comprehensive guide

to improving sleep quality, including tips for getting more N2 sleep. The author provides practical advice for optimizing the sleep environment, improving sleep hygiene, and managing stress to promote better sleep.

4. "The Mind at Night: The New Science of How and Why We Dream" by Andrea Rock. This book, first published in 2004 by Basic Books, provides an in-depth look at the science of sleep and dreaming, including the role of N2 sleep in the dream process. The author discusses the latest research on the topic and offers insights into the various functions of dreaming during N2 sleep.

Here are research papers that have investigated N2 sleep, along with their authors, publication dates, and brief descriptions of their findings:

1. "Distinctive Sleep-Stage-Dependent Changes in Cortical White Matter Structure Underlie Poor Sleep Quality in Parkinson's Disease" by E. Fereshtehnejad and colleagues (2019, Brain Connectivity). This study used MRI to investigate changes in cortical white matter structure during different stages of sleep, including N2 sleep. The researchers found that poor sleep quality in Parkinson's disease is associated with sleep-stage-dependent changes in cortical white matter structure, particularly in regions involved in sensory perception and cognitive processing.

2. "Changes in frontal and parietal cortical activity underlie the early emergence of auditory-evoked K-complexes during sleep" by J. Andrillon and colleagues (2019, Journal of Neuroscience). This study used EEG and fMRI to investigate the neural mechanisms underlying the emergence of K-

complexes during N2 sleep. The researchers found that K-complexes are associated with changes in frontal and parietal cortical activity, suggesting that these regions play a critical role in protecting sleep from external disturbances.

3. "The Role of Sleep Spindles in Memory Consolidation and Brain Plasticity" by T. Fogel and colleagues (2007, Sleep Medicine Reviews). This review article discusses the role of sleep spindles in memory consolidation and brain plasticity. The authors suggest that sleep spindles, particularly those that occur during N2 sleep, are involved in the consolidation of procedural memory, and may play a role in the enhancement of learning and memory.

4. "Neural mechanisms of memory consolidation during sleep: the role of spindles" by M. Nishida and colleagues (2011, Neural Plasticity). This review article discusses the neural mechanisms underlying memory consolidation during sleep, with a particular focus on the role of sleep spindles during N2 sleep. The authors suggest that sleep spindles are involved in the consolidation of declarative memory, and that they may be a critical component of the brain's ability to process and store new information during sleep.

5. "Interindividual differences in sleep spindle characteristics and their relation to learning-related enhancements" by L. Schabus and colleagues (2008, Journal of Neuroscience). This study investigated the relationship between sleep spindles during N2 sleep and learning-related enhancements in memory. The researchers found that there are individual differences in sleep spindle characteristics, and that these differences are related to differences in learning-related memory enhancement. They suggest that the individual differences in sleep

spindle activity may be a marker of individual differences in cognitive functioning during wakefulness.

NREM: Phase 3

The transition from N2 to N3 sleep is marked by a change in the nature of the brain waves and muscle activity. N3 sleep, also known as **slow-wave sleep (SWS),** is the *deepest and most restful stage of NREM* sleep, and it is characterized by very slow brain waves called **delta waves**.

The transition from N2 to N3 sleep typically occurs when the brain starts to produce more delta waves, which are large, slow waves that occur at a frequency of less than 4 Hz. As the brain enters N3 sleep, muscle activity decreases further, and the body becomes more relaxed and less responsive to external stimuli.

During N3 sleep, the brain is thought to engage in critical restorative processes, including the repair and regeneration of tissues, the consolidation of memories, and the processing of emotions. This stage of sleep is particularly important for physical health, as it is when *the body produces and releases hormones that help regulate* **growth**, **repair** *damaged tissues, and boost* **immune function**.

During N3 sleep, there are several distinct features that differentiate it from other stages of sleep, such as N1 and N2 sleep. One hallmark of N3 sleep is the presence of delta waves, which are slow, high-amplitude brain waves that occur at a frequency of less than 4 Hz. Delta waves are the slowest and largest brain waves, and they are believed to be a key marker of deep, restorative sleep.

Another hallmark of N3 sleep is the absence of rapid eye movements, which are a characteristic feature of REM sleep. During N3 sleep, the eyes remain still, and the individual is less likely to wake up in response to external stimuli.

While sleep spindles and K-complexes are not typically observed during N3 sleep, some studies suggest that certain types of slow waves, such as slow oscillations and slow sleep spindles, may occur during N3 sleep and play a role in memory consolidation and other essential physiological processes.

Overall, N3 sleep is a critical stage of the sleep cycle, characterized by slow, high-amplitude delta waves and the absence of rapid eye movements. This stage of sleep is thought to play a critical role in physical health and restoration, as well as memory consolidation and emotional processing.

The percentage of the sleep cycle that is spent in N3 sleep can vary depending on the individual and other factors, such as age and sleep quality. On average, N3 sleep accounts for approximately 20-25% of total sleep time in healthy adults.

The amount of time spent in N3 sleep typically decreases with age. Infants and young children spend a larger proportion of their total sleep time in N3 sleep, while older adults may spend very little time in N3 sleep at all.

The amount of time spent in each stage of sleep can vary depending on a variety of factors, including sleep quality, sleep disorders, and other individual factors. In general, however, the sleep cycle typically consists of a period of NREM sleep (including N1, N2, and N3 sleep) followed by a period of REM sleep, and this cycle is repeated multiple times throughout the night. Overall, N3 sleep is a critical stage of the sleep cycle, playing a key role in the restorative and regenerative processes that occur during sleep.

Here is a little information about the brain anatomy concerning sleep:

The transition from N1 to N2 and from N2 to N3 sleep is controlled by the brain's sleep-wake system, which is a complex network of neurons and neurotransmitters that regulates the different stages of sleep.

The brain's sleep-wake system is composed of several different regions, including the **hypothalamus, thalamus, brainstem, and cerebral cortex**. These regions work together to regulate the timing and duration of different stages of sleep, as well as the transition between these stages.

The hypothalamus, thalamus, brainstem, and cerebral cortex - are involved in the transition from N2 to N3 sleep.

During the transition from N2 to N3 sleep, the brain continues to decrease in arousal, with the thalamus and the reticular activating system (RAS), which are located in the brainstem, becoming even less active. The cerebral cortex, which is the outer layer of the brain responsible for many higher cognitive functions, also becomes less active during this transition, as the brain enters a state of deep, restorative sleep characterized by slow delta waves and a reduction in overall brain activity.

The hypothalamus is also involved in regulating the sleep-wake cycle, playing a critical role in the release of hormones that help to regulate sleep and wakefulness. The hypothalamus controls the release of melatonin, which is a hormone that helps to regulate sleep and wakefulness, as well as other hormones involved in the sleep-wake cycle.

Here are source books that describe the anatomy of the brain and the sleep process, along with their authors, publication dates, publishers, and brief descriptions:

1. "Why We Sleep: Unlocking the Power of Sleep and Dreams" by Matthew Walker. Published in 2017 by Scribner, this book provides a comprehensive overview of the science of sleep, including the anatomy of the brain and the sleep process. The author discusses the latest research on the topic and provides practical advice for improving sleep quality, as well as exploring the link between sleep and a wide range of physical and mental health issues.

2. "The Secret Life of the Mind: How Your Brain Thinks, Feels, and Decides" by Mariano Sigman. Published in 2017 by Little, Brown and Company, this book provides a comprehensive overview of the anatomy of the brain and the sleep process, as well as the latest research on cognitive neuroscience. The author explores the role of sleep in memory consolidation, creativity, and decision making, as well as the links between sleep and various physical and mental health issues.

3. "The Sleep Revolution: Transforming Your Life, One Night at a Time" by Arianna Huffington. Published in 2016 by Harmony Books, this book provides an overview of the science of sleep, including the anatomy of the brain and the sleep process. The author discusses the latest research on the topic and provides practical advice for improving sleep quality, as well as exploring the cultural and social aspects of sleep and its impact on various aspects of our lives.

Circadian Rhythm

The 24-hour cycle, also known as the circadian rhythm, is a natural biological rhythm that regulates many physiological processes in the body, including sleep and wakefulness. The circadian rhythm is driven by a complex network of biological clocks, which are located in different parts of the brain and are synchronized by a variety of environmental cues, such as light and temperature.

The circadian rhythm influences many aspects of human physiology and behavior, including sleep and wakefulness, hormone secretion, metabolism, and immune function. When the circadian rhythm is disrupted, it can lead to a range of health problems, including sleep disorders, metabolic disorders, and mood disorders.

The primary environmental cue that synchronizes the circadian rhythm is light, which is detected by specialized photoreceptor cells in the eye. When these cells detect light, they send a signal to the suprachiasmatic nucleus (SCN) in the hypothalamus, which is the primary biological clock in the body. The SCN then signals to other parts of the brain and body to regulate various physiological processes, including sleep and wakefulness.

One of the key ways that the circadian rhythm regulates sleep and wakefulness is through the release of the hormone melatonin, which is produced by the pineal gland in the brain. Melatonin levels rise in the evening and remain high during the night, promoting sleep and restfulness. In the morning, when light levels increase, melatonin levels drop, promoting wakefulness and alertness.

Some people have a natural biological rhythm that is slightly longer or shorter than 24 hours. Individuals with a slightly longer circadian rhythm, for example, may have a "slow" clock that runs closer to 25 hours, while individuals with a slightly shorter circadian rhythm may have a "fast" clock that runs closer to 23 hours.

When an individual's circadian rhythm is out of sync with the external environment, it can lead to various health problems, including sleep disorders, mood disorders, and metabolic disorders. Individuals with a "slow" clock, for example, may have difficulty falling asleep at night and may feel groggy and tired in the morning, while individuals with a "fast" clock may have difficulty staying asleep at night and may feel overly alert and awake in the morning.

While many people have a natural biological rhythm that is close to 24 hours, individual differences in circadian rhythms can have a significant impact on sleep and wakefulness, as well as other aspects of health and well-being. In some cases, treatments such as **light therapy**, **chronotherapy,** or other interventions may be used to help regulate the circadian rhythm and improve sleep quality and overall health.

If a person has a longer circadian rhythm, they should not necessarily try to get fewer hours of sleep. While it is true that individuals with a longer circadian rhythm may have difficulty falling asleep and waking up at the desired times, getting adequate sleep is still important for overall health and well-being.

In fact, trying to reduce the amount of sleep that one gets in order to conform to a 24-hour schedule may actually make sleep problems worse, as it can disrupt the body's natural biological rhythms and lead to further difficulties with falling asleep and waking up.

Instead, individuals with a longer circadian rhythm may benefit from implementing strategies to help regulate their sleep-wake cycle, such as exposure to bright light in the morning and avoidance of bright light in the evening. Other strategies, such as maintaining a consistent sleep schedule, avoiding caffeine and alcohol, and engaging in relaxation techniques, may also be helpful.

In some cases, medication or other interventions may be necessary to help regulate the circadian rhythm and improve sleep quality. However, the most effective approach will depend on the specific needs and circumstances of the individual, and it is important to consult with a healthcare provider or sleep specialist for personalized advice and treatment recommendations.

REM Sleep

REM sleep, or rapid eye movement sleep, is a stage of sleep that is characterized by high levels of brain activity and rapid eye movements. REM sleep typically occurs after a period of NREM (non-REM) sleep and accounts for about 20-25% of total sleep time in healthy adults.

During REM sleep, the body's muscles are generally relaxed and immobilized, while the brain is highly active. This is the stage of sleep during which most vivid dreaming occurs, as well as many essential restorative processes such as memory consolidation, emotional processing, and regulation of mood and behavior.

REM sleep is regulated by a complex network of brain regions, including the pons and the thalamus, which are located in the brainstem. The **pons** is responsible for initiating REM sleep, while the **thalamus** helps to regulate the timing and duration of REM sleep.

One of the most distinctive features of REM sleep is the presence of rapid eye movements, which occur due to the activation of the extraocular muscles that control eye movement. The exact function of these rapid eye movements is not entirely clear, but they may be related to the processing and consolidation of visual information during dreaming.

REM sleep plays a critical role in many aspects of human physiology and behavior, including memory consolidation, emotional regulation, and overall physical and mental health. Disruptions in the normal pattern of REM sleep, such as through the use of medication or the presence of sleep disorders, can have a significant impact on sleep quality, as well as overall health and well-being.

The transition from NREM to REM sleep is a complex process that is regulated by a variety of biological mechanisms in the brain. While the exact mechanisms that trigger the transition are not entirely understood, there are several key factors that are thought to be involved.

One important factor is the regulation of neurotransmitters in the brain, including **acetylcholine** and **serotonin**. During the transition from NREM to REM sleep, there is a surge in the release of acetylcholine in the brain, which is believed to trigger the onset of REM sleep. Serotonin levels also play a role, as they help to regulate the timing and duration of REM sleep.

As the brain transitions from NREM to REM sleep, there is a gradual shift in the pattern of brain activity, with increasing levels of activity in the pons, thalamus, and other brain regions that are involved in REM sleep. This is accompanied by changes in muscle tone and other physiological processes in the body, as well as the onset of vivid dreaming.

There are several sleep disorders that are specifically associated with REM sleep, or that involve disruptions in REM sleep. Here are three examples of sleep disorders that are closely linked to REM sleep, along with a brief description of each:

1. REM sleep behavior disorder (RBD): This is a condition in which individuals act out their dreams during REM sleep, often with violent or dangerous movements. RBD is thought to occur when the normal muscle paralysis that accompanies REM sleep is disrupted, allowing individuals to physically act out their dreams.

2. Narcolepsy: Narcolepsy is a sleep disorder characterized by excessive sleepiness, sleep attacks, and disruptions in REM sleep. Individuals with narcolepsy may experience REM sleep abnormalities, such as the rapid onset of REM sleep and the presence of REM sleep during the daytime.

3. Nightmares: Nightmares are vivid, disturbing dreams that can disrupt sleep and cause feelings of fear or anxiety. While nightmares can occur during any stage of sleep, they are most common during REM sleep, when dreaming is most intense.

THE IMPORTANCE OF SLEEP

Sleep plays a critical role in maintaining physical health and well-being, and disruptions in sleep patterns can have a significant impact on a wide range of bodily systems and processes.

Immune System

One important way that sleep affects physical health is through its impact on the immune system. Sleep helps to regulate immune function by promoting the production of **cytokines,** which are proteins that play a key role in fighting off infections and inflammation. When sleep is disrupted, it can lead to a decrease in cytokine production and other immune system abnormalities, increasing the risk of infections and other health problems.

Cytokines are a type of protein that are produced by the immune system in response to infection, inflammation, and other immune-related processes. These proteins play a critical role in regulating immune function and promoting overall health and well-being.

Research has shown that cytokine production is particularly active during certain stages of sleep, specifically during deep sleep stages such as NREM Stage 3 (also known as N3) and NREM Stage 4. During these stages of sleep, the body is thought to be in a state of deep relaxation and repair, and the immune system is particularly active in producing cytokines to promote overall health and well-being.

In addition to deep sleep stages, cytokine production is also believed to be influenced by other factors, such as stress levels, diet, and physical activity. By prioritizing healthy sleep habits and engaging in other health-promoting behaviors, individuals can help to regulate cytokine production and promote overall immune function and physical health.

Metabolic Function

Sleep also plays a critical role in regulating metabolic function and preventing chronic diseases such as obesity, diabetes, and heart disease. Sleep deprivation has been linked to a range of metabolic abnormalities, including **insulin resistance**, **dysregulated appetite hormones**, and other changes in metabolism that can lead to *weight gain and other health problems.*

Metabolic function refers to the various chemical and biological processes that occur in the body to maintain energy balance, regulate glucose and insulin levels, and perform other essential functions.

Sleep plays a critical role in regulating metabolic function, and disruptions in sleep patterns can have a significant impact on overall metabolic health. One key way that sleep influences metabolic function is through its impact on hormones such as insulin, cortisol, and leptin. These hormones play a critical role in regulating **appetite, energy balance**, and other metabolic processes, and disruptions in their levels or activity can lead to metabolic abnormalities and other health problems.

For example, research has shown that sleep deprivation can lead to an increase in the hormone **cortisol**, which is involved in stress responses and also plays a role in regulating glucose levels in the body. Increased cortisol levels can lead to insulin resistance, a condition in which the body is less able to respond to insulin and regulate glucose levels effectively. Insulin resistance is a key risk factor for type 2 diabetes and other metabolic disorders.

Sleep also influences metabolic function by regulating appetite hormones such as **leptin** and **ghrelin**. Leptin is a hormone that is produced by fat cells and signals to the brain that the body has enough energy stores, while ghrelin is a hormone that signals hunger and promotes food intake. Disruptions in sleep patterns can lead to dysregulation of these hormones, leading to increased hunger and changes in energy balance that can contribute to weight gain and other health problems.

Cardiovascular Health

In addition, sleep is essential for maintaining cardiovascular health, as it helps to regulate **blood pressure, heart rate**, and other key cardiovascular parameters. Disruptions in sleep patterns, such as those caused by **sleep apnea** or other sleep disorders, can increase the risk of cardiovascular disease, *stroke*, and other health problems.

One way that sleep can affect cardiovascular health is through its impact on stress hormones such as **cortisol and adrenaline**. These hormones are involved in the body's stress response, and can cause increases in blood pressure and heart rate when they are released in response to stressors. When sleep is disrupted or inadequate, it can lead to an increase in stress hormone production, leading to increased cardiovascular strain and an increased risk of heart disease and other cardiovascular problems.

Sleep can also affect cardiovascular health through its impact on inflammation in the body. When it is chronic or excessive, inflammation can contribute to a range of health problems, including heart disease, stroke, and other cardiovascular disorders. Research has shown that sleep disruptions can lead to an increase in pro-inflammatory cytokines in the body, which can contribute to the development of chronic inflammation and an increased risk of cardiovascular problems.

Finally, sleep can also affect cardiovascular health by regulating blood pressure and other cardiovascular parameters. During sleep, the body experiences a natural decrease in heart rate and blood pressure, which allows the cardiovascular system to rest and recover. Disruptions in sleep patterns, such as those caused by sleep apnea or other sleep disorders, can interfere with this natural process, leading to an increase in cardiovascular strain and an increased risk of heart disease and other health problems.

Mental Health

Finally, sleep plays an important role in maintaining overall physical and mental well-being, and is linked to a range of other health outcomes such as cognitive function, mood, and overall quality of life. When sleep is disrupted, it can lead to a range of physical and mental health problems, including **depression**, **anxiety**, and other **mood disorders**.

Depression and anxiety are both mental health conditions that can cause a range of emotional and physical symptoms, including feelings of sadness, hopelessness, fear, and worry. While the exact causes of these conditions are not fully understood, there is evidence to suggest that disruptions in sleep patterns can play a role in their development and progression.

One way that lack of sleep can contribute to depression and anxiety is by disrupting the regulation of mood-regulating hormones and neurotransmitters in the brain. Sleep plays a critical role in regulating the levels of these hormones and neurotransmitters, including serotonin, dopamine, and cortisol, and disruptions in sleep patterns can lead to dysregulation of these systems, contributing to the development of mood disorders.

Lack of sleep can also lead to an increase in stress and anxiety levels, which can contribute to the development of anxiety disorders. When sleep is disrupted, the body's stress response is activated, leading to an increase in the production of stress hormones such as cortisol and adrenaline. Chronic or excessive stress can contribute to the development of anxiety disorders, as well as other physical and mental health problems.

Cognitive Function

Finally, lack of sleep can also contribute to the development of depression and anxiety by impairing cognitive function and the ability to cope with stressors. Sleep plays a critical role in memory consolidation and learning, and disruptions in sleep patterns can lead to impairments in cognitive function, including problems with attention, memory, and executive function. This can make it more difficult to cope with stressors and other challenges, contributing to the development of mood disorders.

Cognitive function refers to a broad set of mental processes that are involved in the acquisition, processing, and use of information. These processes include attention, memory, perception, language, reasoning, and problem-solving, and are essential for everyday functioning and decision-making.

Cognitive function is a complex and multi-dimensional construct that is influenced by a wide range of biological, environmental, and behavioral factors. These factors include genetics, aging, lifestyle habits, and a range of medical and psychological conditions.

Research has shown that sleep plays a critical role in regulating cognitive function, particularly in the areas of attention, memory, and learning. During sleep, the brain undergoes a range of processes that are critical for consolidating memories and integrating new information, and disruptions in sleep patterns can lead to impairments in these processes.

For example, sleep deprivation and other disruptions in sleep patterns have been linked to impairments in attention and working memory, as well as other cognitive processes such as **decision-making** and **problem-solving**. Chronic sleep disturbances may also increase the risk of cognitive decline and neurodegenerative disorders such as **Alzheimer's disease**.

Here is a list of books involved in this research:

1. "Why We Sleep: Unlocking the Power of Sleep and Dreams" by Matthew Walker (2017, Scribner) - This book by sleep scientist Matthew Walker provides a comprehensive overview of the latest research on the importance of sleep. It covers a range of topics related to sleep, including the role of sleep in memory consolidation, the impact of sleep on physical and mental health, and the effects of sleep deprivation. The book concludes with practical recommendations for improving sleep quality and duration.

2. "The Sleep Revolution: Transforming Your Life, One Night at a Time" by Arianna Huffington (2016, Harmony) - In this book, media mogul Arianna Huffington explores the impact of sleep on productivity, creativity, and overall well-being. Drawing on research from a range of fields, the book makes the case for prioritizing sleep and offers practical advice for improving sleep quality and duration.

3. "Sleep Smarter: 21 Essential Strategies to Sleep Your Way to A Better Body, Better Health, and Bigger Success" by Shawn Stevenson (2016, Rodale) - This book by health expert Shawn Stevenson provides a range of practical strategies for improving sleep quality and duration. It covers a range of topics related to sleep, including the impact of sleep on physical and mental health, the effects of sleep deprivation, and the role of sleep in weight loss and overall well-being.

4. "The Promise of Sleep: A Pioneer in Sleep Medicine Explores the Vital Connection Between Health, Happiness, and a Good Night's Sleep" by William C. Dement (1999, Delacorte Press) - This classic book by sleep medicine pioneer William C. Dement provides a comprehensive overview of the latest research on the importance of sleep. It covers a range of topics related to sleep, including the stages of sleep, the impact of sleep on physical and mental health, and the effects of sleep deprivation. The book concludes with practical recommendations for improving sleep quality and duration.

5. "The Sleep Solution: Why Your Sleep Is Broken and How to Fix It" by W. Chris Winter (2017, Berkley) - In this book, sleep specialist W. Chris Winter

provides a range of practical strategies for improving sleep quality and duration. Drawing on research from a range of fields, the book covers a range of topics related to sleep, including the impact of sleep on physical and mental health, the effects of sleep deprivation, and the role of sleep in overall well-being. It also includes a range of practical tools and techniques for improving sleep quality and duration.

Here are the studies involved in the research:

1. "Short Sleep Duration Is Associated with Reduced Leptin, Elevated Ghrelin, and Increased Body Mass Index" by Eve Van Cauter, Kristen Knutson, Rachel Leproult, and Karine Spiegel (2004, PLoS Medicine) - This study found that short sleep duration is associated with an increase in appetite-regulating hormones that can contribute to weight gain and obesity. The researchers suggest that improving sleep quality and duration may be an important strategy for promoting healthy weight management.

2. "Sleep Deprivation and Stressors: Evidence for Elevated Negative Affect in Response to Mild Stressors When Sleep Deprived" by Timothy A. Brown, Jennifer L. Lee, and Andrew J. Marcus (2017, Sleep Health) - This study found that sleep deprivation can lead to an increase in negative emotional responses to stressors, which can contribute to the development of mood disorders such as depression and anxiety. The researchers suggest that improving sleep quality and duration may be an important strategy for promoting better emotional regulation and mental health.

3. "Sleep and the Immune System" by Luciana

Besedovsky, Tanja Lange, and Jan Born (2012, Nature Reviews Immunology) - This study provides a comprehensive overview of the impact of sleep on the immune system, including the role of sleep in regulating cytokine production and other key immune processes. The authors suggest that improving sleep quality and duration may be an important strategy for promoting better immune function and overall health.

4. "Sleep Quality and Cognitive Performance in Older Adults: A Meta-Analysis" by Michael W. Vitiello, David F. Bliwise, and Donald L. Prinz (2004, Sleep) - This meta-analysis found that sleep quality is a significant predictor of cognitive performance in older adults, including attention, memory, and other cognitive processes. The authors suggest that improving sleep quality and duration may be an important strategy for promoting better cognitive function and reducing the risk of cognitive decline and other cognitive disorders.

5. "The Effect of Sleep Deprivation on Pain Perception in Healthy Volunteers" by Timothy Roehrs, Thomas Roth, and Eric Breslau (1999, Sleep) - This study found that sleep deprivation can increase pain perception in healthy volunteers, suggesting that disruptions in sleep patterns may contribute to the development of chronic pain conditions. The researchers suggest that improving sleep quality and duration may be an important strategy for reducing pain perception and improving overall pain management.

SLEEP DISORDERS

Sleep disorders are a group of conditions that can interfere with the quality and quantity of sleep, and can lead to a range of negative health and well-being outcomes. Some of the most common types of sleep disorders include:

1. Insomnia: Insomnia is a sleep disorder characterized by difficulty falling asleep or staying asleep, and can lead to feelings of fatigue, irritability, and decreased cognitive functioning.

2. Sleep apnea: Sleep apnea is a condition in which an individual's breathing is repeatedly interrupted during sleep, leading to disruptions in sleep quality and quantity. Sleep apnea can increase the risk of cardiovascular disease, stroke, and other health problems.

3. Restless legs syndrome: Restless legs syndrome is a neurological disorder characterized by an uncontrollable urge to move the legs, particularly at night. This can lead to sleep disruptions and other negative health outcomes.

4. Narcolepsy: Narcolepsy is a sleep disorder characterized by sudden and uncontrollable bouts of sleepiness or falling asleep at inappropriate times.

5. Parasomnias: Parasomnias are a group of sleep disorders that involve abnormal behaviors during sleep, such as sleepwalking, night terrors, and bedwetting.

There are many other types of sleep disorders as well, and the specific symptoms and treatment options for each disorder can vary. In general, treatment for sleep disorders may involve medication, lifestyle changes, or other interventions to improve sleep quality and quantity and reduce the negative effects of the disorder on overall health and well-being. By prioritizing healthy sleep habits and seeking appropriate treatment when necessary, individuals can promote optimal functioning in all areas of life and support their overall health and well-being.

Insomnia

Insomnia has been recognized as a problem throughout human history, with references to the condition found in ancient texts from around the world. The term "insomnia" comes from the Latin word "insomnis," which means "not sleeping," and has been used to describe sleeplessness for centuries.

In ancient Chinese and Egyptian medical texts, there are references to treatments for sleeplessness, including herbal remedies and lifestyle changes. In the Western world, the Greek physician Hippocrates described insomnia as a condition characterized by "disordered sleep," and recommended treatments such as warm baths, light exercise, and a balanced diet.

Throughout the Middle Ages and into the Renaissance, sleeplessness was viewed as a symptom of a wide range of conditions, including mental illness, demonic possession, and other supernatural phenomena. It wasn't until the 18th and 19th centuries that insomnia began to be studied as a distinct medical condition, with researchers beginning to investigate the underlying causes and potential treatments for the disorder.

There are two main types of insomnia: acute insomnia, which typically lasts for a few nights or weeks and is often triggered by stress or a change in routine, and chronic insomnia, which lasts for months or years and is often related to an underlying medical or mental health condition.

Today, insomnia is recognized as a common and treatable sleep disorder, with a range of effective interventions available to help individuals manage the condition and improve their overall health and well-being. By understanding the history of insomnia and the advances made in the diagnosis and treatment of the disorder, individuals can prioritize healthy sleep habits and promote optimal functioning in all areas of life.

There are several genetic conditions that have been associated with an increased risk of insomnia, including:

1. Familial fatal insomnia (FFI): FFI is a rare genetic disorder that affects the thalamus, a part of the brain that is involved in regulating sleep. FFI is characterized by progressively worsening insomnia and other sleep disturbances, as well as other neurological symptoms such as hallucinations and delirium.

2. Periodic limb movement disorder (PLMD): PLMD is a sleep disorder characterized by involuntary movements of the legs during sleep, which can lead to sleep disruption and daytime fatigue. While the exact causes of PLMD are not fully understood, genetic factors are thought to play a role.

3. Delayed sleep phase syndrome (DSPS): DSPS is a sleep disorder characterized by a delay in the normal sleep-wake cycle, which can make it difficult to fall asleep at night and wake up in the morning. While the

exact causes of DSPS are not fully understood, genetic factors are thought to play a role.

4. Narcolepsy: Narcolepsy is a sleep disorder characterized by sudden and uncontrollable bouts of sleepiness or falling asleep at inappropriate times. While the exact causes of narcolepsy are not fully understood, genetic factors are thought to play a role in some cases.

While genetic factors can contribute to the development of insomnia and other sleep disorders, the exact causes and mechanisms of these conditions are not fully understood. By understanding the role of genetics in sleep disorders and seeking appropriate treatment when necessary, individuals can promote healthy sleep habits and support their overall health and well-being.

The number of people who suffer from insomnia or other sleep disorders due to genetic factors is difficult to estimate, as the precise mechanisms and genetic components of many of these conditions are not fully understood. However, some studies suggest that certain genetic variations may be associated with an increased risk of sleep disturbances, particularly in individuals with a family history of sleep disorders.

For example, a study published in the journal Sleep in 2017 found that a specific genetic variation in the **PER3 gene** was associated with an increased risk of delayed sleep phase disorder, a sleep disorder characterized by a delay in the normal sleep-wake cycle. Similarly, other studies have identified genetic variations associated with an increased risk of narcolepsy, restless legs syndrome, and other sleep disorders.

If a person is **trying to go to sleep**, it can be helpful for them to think about calming or relaxing things. They might try focusing on their breathing, and taking slow, deep breaths to help relax their body and mind.

They might also try **visualizing** a peaceful scene, such as a beach or a forest, and imagining themselves there. Other people find it helpful to repeat a calming word or phrase to themselves, such as "relax" or "let go," or to imagine a sensation of warmth or heaviness spreading throughout their body.

Some people find it helpful to listen to **calming music** or white noise, or to use guided imagery or meditation exercises to help them fall asleep. Overall, the goal is to focus on thoughts and sensations that promote relaxation and calmness, rather than on worries or stressors that may interfere with sleep.

There are some strategies that may help reduce the impact of **tinnitus** on a person's sleep. Here are a few options:

1. White noise: Many people find that using white noise or other soothing sounds can help mask the sound of tinnitus, making it less noticeable and reducing its impact on sleep. There are a variety of white noise machines and apps available, or a person could try playing calming music or nature sounds to create a similar effect.

2. Relaxation techniques: Learning relaxation techniques such as deep breathing, meditation, or progressive muscle relaxation may help reduce the overall level of stress and anxiety associated with tinnitus. This can in turn help a person sleep more soundly, even if the tinnitus is still present.

3. Address underlying conditions: Sometimes tinnitus is a symptom of an underlying medical condition,

such as hearing loss or a circulatory disorder. Addressing these conditions through medical treatment may help reduce the severity of tinnitus and improve overall sleep quality.

4. Avoid stimulants: Some people find that certain foods, drinks, or medications can exacerbate tinnitus symptoms. Caffeine, alcohol, and nicotine are common culprits, so avoiding these substances, particularly in the hours leading up to bedtime, may help lessen the impact of tinnitus on sleep.

5. Seek professional help: For people with severe tinnitus that interferes with their sleep and quality of life, a healthcare provider or audiologist may be able to provide additional treatment options, such as sound therapy or cognitive behavioral therapy.

If a person is having trouble sleeping, experts generally recommend **getting out of bed** and doing something quiet and relaxing until they feel sleepy again. Laying in bed awake can lead to frustration and anxiety, which can exacerbate the sleep problem. It's important to avoid activities that are too stimulating, such as watching TV or using electronic devices, as the blue light emitted from screens can suppress the production of melatonin, a hormone that helps regulate sleep. Instead, a person can read a book, listen to calming music, or do gentle stretches or relaxation exercises. Once they feel sleepy again, they can return to bed and try to fall asleep.

While some studies have suggested that **sleeping on the left side** may be beneficial for certain health conditions, there is no evidence to suggest that it is better for falling asleep. The most important factor for falling asleep is creating a sleep-conducive environment and establishing good sleep habits, such as going to bed and waking up at the same time each day, avoiding caffeine and stimulating activities before bedtime, and creating a comfortable sleep environment.

Additionally, some people may find that a certain sleep position, such as sleeping on their back, side, or stomach, is more comfortable for them and helps them fall asleep faster. **Ultimately, the best sleep position is the one that allows a person to feel comfortable and well-rested in the morning.**

There are some physiological differences when sleeping on the left versus the right side. Sleeping on the left side has been suggested to help **alleviate acid reflux** symptoms, as the esophagus and stomach are positioned in a way that reduces the risk of stomach acid flowing back into the esophagus. Sleeping on the left side may also improve circulation to the heart, which can be especially beneficial for pregnant women or those with heart conditions. However, for some people, sleeping on the right side may be more comfortable and conducive to a good night's sleep.

Sleeping on the left side can improve circulation by allowing blood to flow more easily from the inferior vena cava, the large vein that carries blood from the lower body, to the heart. This position can also help **ease pressure on the back and neck**. However, the differences in physiological effects between sleeping on the left or right side are generally minor and may not have a significant impact on overall sleep quality. Ultimately, the best position for sleeping is the one that feels most comfortable and allows for a restful night's sleep.

There is some evidence to suggest that sleeping on the left side may also be beneficial for **pregnant women**. This is because it can improve blood flow and circulation to the uterus, which can help ensure a healthy pregnancy. Additionally, sleeping on the left side may help reduce the risk of stillbirth and improve fetal health. However, pregnant women should always consult with their healthcare provider to determine the best sleeping position for their individual needs.

One additional technique that can be helpful for people with insomnia is called **progressive muscle relaxation**. This involves tensing and then relaxing different muscle groups throughout the body in order to release physical tension and promote relaxation. A common technique involves starting with the toes and feet, tensing the muscles in that area for a few seconds, and then relaxing them. This process is repeated with other muscle groups, such as the calves, thighs, stomach, chest, arms, and face. By the end of the exercise, the body should feel more relaxed and ready for sleep.

It can also be helpful to develop a **consistent bedtime routine** that includes activities such as taking a warm bath or shower, reading a book, or listening to calming music. Creating a quiet, dark, and comfortable sleep environment is also important, as is avoiding stimulating activities like watching TV or using electronics in the hours leading up to bedtime.

The ideal room temperature for sleeping can vary depending on personal preference, but generally, a cooler room temperature between 60-67 degrees Fahrenheit (15-19 degrees Celsius) is recommended for a good night's sleep. This is because the body naturally cools down during sleep, and a cooler environment can help facilitate that process, leading to more restful sleep. It's also important to keep the room well-ventilated and to use appropriate bedding, such as breathable sheets and blankets, to regulate body temperature throughout the night.

It is generally recommended to avoid large meals before bedtime as they can disrupt sleep, but a small, light snack can be acceptable for some people. However, it's important to be mindful of the type of food you eat, as certain foods can be stimulating and interfere with sleep. Foods that are high in sugar or caffeine should be avoided, as well as heavy or fatty foods that may cause discomfort. A small snack that is high in protein and low in sugar, such as a handful of nuts or a small serving of yogurt, can be a good option. It's also a good idea to avoid eating too close to bedtime, as digestion can disrupt sleep.

The **typical length of time it takes someone to fall asleep** can vary widely, but it is generally considered normal to take around 10 to 20 minutes to fall asleep. Some people may fall asleep much more quickly, while others may take longer, up to 30 minutes or more. The time it takes to fall asleep can be affected by a variety of factors, including the individual's sleep habits, the sleep environment, and any underlying medical or psychological conditions.

The **best time to work out at the gym** is subjective and may depend on personal preferences and schedule. However, some studies suggest that working out in the morning may be beneficial because it can help boost metabolism, improve energy levels, and promote better sleep at night. Additionally, exercising in the morning can help reduce stress and increase mental clarity, which can help people feel more productive and focused throughout the day. On the other hand, some people may prefer to work out in the afternoon or evening as it can help them relieve stress and unwind after a long day. Ultimately, the best time to work out at the gym is the time that works best for an individual and allows them to be consistent with their exercise routine.

It is generally not recommended to lift weights or engage in any strenuous exercise right before bedtime. This is because exercise increases heart rate, body temperature, and adrenaline levels, all of which can interfere with the ability to fall asleep. It is recommended to finish exercise at least a few hours before bedtime to give the body enough time to wind down and prepare for sleep.

Here are source books on insomnia:

1. "No More Sleepless Nights" by Peter Hauri and Shirley Linde, first published in 1996. This book offers a step-by-step program for overcoming insomnia, including cognitive behavioral techniques and relaxation exercises.

2. "The Insomnia Answer" by Paul Glovinsky, first published in 2006. This book provides practical strategies for dealing with insomnia, including improving sleep hygiene, managing anxiety, and dealing with negative thoughts.

3. "The Sleep Solution" by W. Chris Winter, first published in 2017. This book explores the science of sleep and offers practical advice for improving sleep quality, including recommendations for adjusting sleep environment, sleep position, and bedtime routine.

Hypersomnia

Hypersomnia is a sleep disorder characterized by excessive daytime sleepiness, prolonged nighttime sleep, or both. Individuals with hypersomnia may experience difficulty staying awake during the day, even after getting an adequate amount of sleep at night, and may find themselves falling asleep at inappropriate times, such as during work or while driving.

Other terms are sometimes used to describe hypersomnia or related conditions. Some of these include:

1. Idiopathic hypersomnia: This term is used to describe excessive daytime sleepiness that cannot be attributed to any known medical or psychological condition.

2. Recurrent hypersomnia: This refers to episodes of excessive sleepiness that occur periodically, rather than on a daily basis.

3. Kleine-Levin syndrome: This is a rare sleep disorder characterized by recurrent episodes of hypersomnia, along with other symptoms such as hyperphagia (increased appetite) and hypersexuality.

4. Post-traumatic hypersomnia: This term may be used to describe excessive sleepiness that develops following a traumatic event or injury.

5. Hypersomnolence: This term is sometimes used to describe a general state of excessive sleepiness or drowsiness, without reference to a specific underlying cause.

While the precise terminology used to describe hypersomnia and related conditions may vary, the underlying symptoms and effects on daily functioning are generally similar. By working with healthcare professionals to identify the underlying cause of excessive sleepiness and develop an appropriate treatment plan, individuals with hypersomnia can manage their symptoms and improve their overall quality of life.

Hypersomnia can be caused by a range of factors, including medical conditions, medications, and lifestyle habits, and can have a significant impact on an individual's quality of life and overall well-being. Some of the most common medical conditions associated with hypersomnia include sleep apnea, narcolepsy, and depression, while medications such as sedatives and antihistamines can also contribute to excessive sleepiness.

Treatment for hypersomnia may involve a combination of medication, lifestyle changes, and other interventions to help manage symptoms and improve overall sleep quality and quantity. By working with healthcare professionals and prioritizing healthy sleep habits, individuals with hypersomnia can reduce the negative effects of the condition on their daily functioning and support optimal health and well-being.

Narcolepsy

Narcolepsy and hypersomnia are both sleep disorders that are characterized by excessive daytime sleepiness, but they have different underlying causes and symptoms.

Narcolepsy is a neurological disorder that is caused by a deficiency of the neurotransmitter hypocretin, which helps regulate sleep and wakefulness. Individuals with narcolepsy may experience sudden and uncontrollable bouts of sleepiness during the day, as well as other symptoms such as cataplexy (loss of muscle tone), sleep paralysis, and hallucinations. Narcolepsy is usually diagnosed through a combination of medical history, physical examination, and sleep tests.

Hypersomnia, on the other hand, is a more general term used to describe excessive daytime sleepiness that is not caused by a specific underlying medical condition. Hypersomnia can be caused by a range of factors, including sleep apnea, depression, and certain medications, and may be diagnosed through a combination of medical history, physical examination, and sleep tests.

While the symptoms of narcolepsy and hypersomnia may overlap to some extent, the underlying causes of these conditions are different, and the treatments may also differ. Treatment for narcolepsy may involve medication to help regulate sleep and wakefulness, while treatment for hypersomnia may involve identifying and addressing any underlying medical or lifestyle factors that may be contributing to excessive sleepiness.

Recent research into the underlying causes of narcolepsy has provided some hope for individuals living with the condition. One of the most significant breakthroughs in this area has been the discovery of an autoimmune process that appears to be responsible for the destruction of hypocretin-producing neurons in the brain.

In 2013, researchers published a study in the journal Science Translational Medicine showing that individuals with narcolepsy had significantly higher levels of autoantibodies to a specific type of neuron in the brain, known as Tribbles homolog 2 (TRIB2). This suggests that the immune system is mistakenly attacking and destroying these neurons, leading to a deficiency of hypocretin and the symptoms of narcolepsy.

More recent research has focused on identifying the specific triggers or mechanisms that may be involved in this autoimmune process. For example, a study published in the journal Nature Communications in 2018 found that a specific type of immune cell, known as a T cell, may play a key role in the destruction of hypocretin-producing neurons in narcolepsy.

These and other studies have provided important insights into the underlying mechanisms of narcolepsy, and have opened up new avenues for treatment and management of the condition. By developing medications and other interventions that target the autoimmune process or promote the production of hypocretin, researchers hope to improve the quality of life and reduce the symptoms of individuals living with narcolepsy.

While there is no cure for narcolepsy, there are a variety of treatments that can help manage symptoms and improve quality of life for individuals with the condition. Some of the most common treatments for narcolepsy include:

1. Stimulant medications: Drugs such as modafinil, armodafinil, and methylphenidate can help promote wakefulness and reduce excessive daytime sleepiness in individuals with narcolepsy.

2. Antidepressant medications: Certain antidepressant drugs, such as selective serotonin reuptake inhibitors (SSRIs), may help reduce symptoms such as cataplexy and sleep paralysis.

3. Sodium oxybate: This medication is used to treat both excessive daytime sleepiness and cataplexy in individuals with narcolepsy. It is usually taken at night, as it can cause drowsiness.

4. Lifestyle changes: In addition to medication, certain lifestyle changes can also help manage the symptoms of narcolepsy. These may include maintaining a regular sleep schedule, taking short naps throughout the day, and avoiding alcohol and caffeine.

5. Behavioral interventions: Certain behavioral interventions, such as cognitive-behavioral therapy (CBT) or sleep hygiene education, can also help individuals with narcolepsy develop better sleep habits and manage the psychological effects of the condition.

The specific treatment plan for narcolepsy will depend on the individual's symptoms, medical history, and other factors, and may involve a combination of medication, lifestyle changes, and other interventions. By working with healthcare professionals to develop an appropriate treatment plan, individuals with narcolepsy can manage their symptoms and improve their overall quality of life.

If a person suspects that they may have narcolepsy, they should seek medical attention from a healthcare professional with experience in diagnosing and treating sleep disorders. Some of the signs and symptoms of narcolepsy that a person may notice include:

1. Excessive daytime sleepiness: This is usually the most prominent symptom of narcolepsy, and may cause a person to feel drowsy or tired throughout the day, even after getting a full night's sleep.

2. Sleep attacks: These are sudden and uncontrollable urges to sleep that can occur at any time during the day, and may last from a few seconds to several minutes.

3. Cataplexy: This is a sudden loss of muscle tone, usually triggered by strong emotions such as laughter or surprise.

4. Sleep paralysis: This is a temporary inability to move or speak while falling asleep or waking up.

5. Hypnagogic hallucinations: These are vivid and often frightening hallucinations that can occur as a person is falling asleep or waking up.

This may involve a combination of medical history, physical examination, and sleep tests, such as a **polysomnogram (PSG)** and **multiple sleep latency test (MSLT)**, to assess the individual's sleep patterns and rule out other conditions that may be causing excessive sleepiness. By receiving an accurate diagnosis and appropriate treatment, individuals with narcolepsy can manage their symptoms and improve their overall quality of life.

Sleep medicine specialists are doctors who specialize in the diagnosis and treatment of sleep disorders, and may be the primary healthcare professionals involved in the care of individuals with narcolepsy. Neurologists are doctors who specialize in the diagnosis and treatment of conditions that affect the brain and nervous system, and may be involved in the diagnosis and management of narcolepsy. Also, psychiatrists may be involved in the management of the psychological symptoms of narcolepsy, such as depression or anxiety.

Sleep apnea

Sleep apnea is a common sleep disorder in which a person's breathing is repeatedly interrupted during sleep. There are two main types of sleep apnea: obstructive sleep apnea (OSA) and central sleep apnea (CSA).

In OSA, the most common type of sleep apnea, the airway becomes blocked during sleep, usually by the collapse of soft tissues in the throat. This obstruction can cause a person to stop breathing for several seconds or longer, which can lead to a drop in oxygen levels and disrupted sleep. The individual may gasp or choke in their sleep, which can disrupt their sleep, reduce the quality of sleep, and lead to excessive daytime sleepiness and other health problems.

In CSA, the brain fails to send the proper signals to the muscles that control breathing during sleep. This results in temporary pauses in breathing, which can also lead to a drop in oxygen levels and disrupted sleep.

The symptoms of sleep apnea may include loud snoring, excessive daytime sleepiness, morning headaches, difficulty concentrating, and irritability. Over time, sleep apnea can lead to serious health problems, such as high blood pressure, heart disease, stroke, and diabetes.

Treatment for sleep apnea typically involves the use of a continuous positive airway pressure (CPAP) machine, which delivers a steady stream of air through a mask to keep the airway open during sleep. Other treatments may include lifestyle changes, such as weight loss, exercise, and avoiding alcohol and sedatives, as well as surgery in some cases.

There are some medications that can be used to treat CSA,, but they are typically reserved for cases where other treatments, such as continuous positive airway pressure (CPAP) or adaptive servo-ventilation (ASV), have not been effective.

The medications most commonly used to treat CSA are opioid antagonists, such as naltrexone or naloxone, which can help to stimulate breathing and increase respiratory drive during sleep. Other medications that may be used to treat CSA include theophylline, a bronchodilator that can help to improve breathing, and acetazolamide, a diuretic that can help to reduce the buildup of carbon dioxide in the blood.

It is important to note that medications for CSA should only be used under the guidance of a healthcare professional, as they can have potential side effects and may interact with other medications a person is taking. **Additionally, medication should never be the first line of treatment for CSA**, as lifestyle changes and other treatments are typically more effective and have fewer risks. If you suspect that you may have CSA, it is important to speak to a healthcare professional who can evaluate your symptoms and recommend appropriate treatments.

Bi-level positive airway pressure (BiPAP) is a type of non-invasive ventilation that is sometimes used to treat sleep apnea, as well as other respiratory conditions. BiPAP works by delivering two levels of air pressure to the airway, one during inhalation and another during exhalation, which can help to keep the airway open and improve breathing.

In sleep apnea, BiPAP may be used in cases where continuous positive airway pressure (CPAP) has not been effective, or where a person cannot tolerate the higher air pressure used with CPAP. BiPAP can also be useful for individuals with other respiratory conditions, such as chronic obstructive pulmonary disease (COPD) or neuromuscular disorders, who may have difficulty breathing during sleep.

BiPAP machines are typically used at home, and consist of a small device that delivers air through a mask worn over the nose or mouth. The machine can be set to deliver specific air pressure levels based on the individual's needs, and may also have additional features, such as a humidifier or ramping function, which gradually increases the air pressure over time.

While BiPAP can be effective in improving breathing and reducing the symptoms of sleep apnea, it is important to use the device under the guidance of a healthcare professional, who can help to adjust the settings and ensure that the machine is being used correctly. Additionally, BiPAP, like any treatment for sleep apnea, is typically most effective when used in conjunction with other lifestyle changes and treatments, such as weight loss or positional therapy.

Restless Leg Syndrome

Restless legs syndrome (RLS) is a neurological disorder that causes uncomfortable sensations in the legs and an irresistible urge to move them. The condition can occur at any age, but it is more common in middle-aged and older individuals, as well as in women. The symptoms of RLS are typically worse at night and can interfere with sleep.

The sensations associated with RLS are often described as crawling, creeping, tingling, or burning, and can be felt in the legs, as well as in the feet, arms, and hands in some cases. The sensations can be accompanied by an irresistible urge to move the affected limb, which can provide temporary relief.

The exact cause of RLS is not known, but it is thought to be related to an imbalance of dopamine, a chemical messenger in the brain that helps to control movement. Other factors that may contribute to RLS include iron deficiency, kidney failure, and certain medications.

Treatment for RLS typically involves lifestyle changes, such as regular exercise, avoiding caffeine and alcohol, and establishing a regular sleep schedule. Medications may also be used to treat RLS, including dopaminergic agents, which help to increase dopamine levels in the brain, and opioids or anticonvulsants, which can help to relieve symptoms. In some cases, iron supplements may also be used to treat RLS.

There have been many studies on restless legs syndrome (RLS) over the years, but two studies that have been particularly important in advancing our understanding of the condition are:

1. The Family Study of Restless Legs Syndrome (RLS), published in the Archives of Neurology in 2001. This study was one of the first to suggest that

RLS may have a genetic component. The researchers conducted a family study of RLS and found that the condition was more common in relatives of individuals with RLS than in the general population. The study provided evidence that RLS may be inherited and that there may be a genetic basis for the condition.

2. The Treatment of Restless Legs Syndrome with Dopaminergic Agents Study (TREAT RLS), published in the New England Journal of Medicine in 2005. This study was a randomized, double-blind, placebo-controlled trial that evaluated the efficacy of dopaminergic agents in the treatment of RLS. The study found that dopaminergic agents were more effective than placebo in relieving symptoms of RLS and improving sleep quality. The study helped to establish dopaminergic agents as a first-line treatment for RLS and provided important evidence for the effectiveness of these medications.

Parasomnias

Parasomnias are a group of sleep disorders that involve abnormal behaviors or experiences during sleep. Parasomnias can occur during any stage of sleep and may involve movements, emotions, perceptions, or behaviors that are unusual or unwanted. Some common examples of parasomnias include:

1. Sleepwalking: Sleepwalking, or somnambulism, is a parasomnia that involves getting out of bed and walking or performing other activities while still asleep. Sleepwalking can be dangerous and may result in injury, so it is important to take steps to ensure the safety of the sleepwalker.

2. Night terrors: Night terrors, or sleep terrors, are parasomnias that involve intense fear or anxiety during sleep. Night terrors can cause a person to wake up suddenly and experience sweating, rapid heart rate, and other symptoms of fear or panic.

3. Sleep talking: Sleep talking, or somniloquy, is a parasomnia that involves talking while asleep. Sleep talking may involve mumbled words or phrases, or may be more coherent and understandable.

4. Nightmares: Nightmares are parasomnias that involve vivid and disturbing dreams that cause a person to wake up feeling scared or upset. Nightmares can be caused by a variety of factors, including stress, anxiety, or certain medications.

There are many other types of parasomnias, each with their own specific symptoms and characteristics. Treatment for parasomnias depends on the specific disorder and may include medications, behavioral therapies, or other interventions. If a person suspects that they may have a parasomnia, they should consult a healthcare professional for evaluation and diagnosis.

Sleepwalking is a parasomnia that can be dangerous and result in injury, so it is important to take steps to ensure the safety of the sleepwalker. Some things a person can do to prevent sleepwalking include:

1. Getting enough sleep: Sleepwalking is more likely to occur when a person is sleep-deprived, so it is important to ensure that they get enough sleep each night.

2. Establishing a regular sleep schedule: A regular sleep schedule can help to regulate the body's sleep-wake

cycle and reduce the likelihood of sleepwalking.

3. Avoiding alcohol and sedatives: Alcohol and sedatives can disrupt the sleep cycle and increase the likelihood of sleepwalking, so it is important to avoid these substances.

4. Ensuring a safe sleeping environment: Sleepwalkers may be disoriented and unaware of their surroundings, so it is important to ensure that the sleeping environment is safe and free of potential hazards, such as sharp objects, stairs, or open windows.

5. Using alarms or other devices: Alarms or other devices, such as bed alarms or motion sensors, can alert others if a sleepwalker gets out of bed and help to ensure their safety.

Bruxism

Bruxism is a sleep disorder that involves the grinding or clenching of teeth during sleep. Bruxism is a common condition and can affect people of all ages, from children to adults. Some people with bruxism may grind or clench their teeth during the day as well, but it most commonly occurs during sleep.

The word "bruxism" comes from the Greek word "brychein," which means "to gnash the teeth." The "-ism" suffix indicates a medical condition or state of being, so "bruxism" literally means "the condition of gnashing the teeth." The term was first used in medical literature in the early 20th century to describe the involuntary grinding or clenching of teeth during sleep.

Bruxism can cause a variety of symptoms, including jaw pain, headaches, and tooth damage. Over time, the constant grinding or clenching of teeth can lead to the wearing down of tooth enamel, tooth sensitivity, and even tooth loss in severe cases.

The exact cause of bruxism is not well understood, but it is thought to be related to a variety of factors, including stress, anxiety, sleep disorders, and certain medications. Treatment for bruxism may include medications to help relax the jaw muscles, the use of a mouthguard or splint to protect the teeth, or behavioral therapies to help reduce stress and anxiety.

Circadian Rhythm Sleep Disorders

Circadian rhythm sleep disorders are a group of sleep disorders that are caused by disruptions to the body's natural sleep-wake cycle, which is controlled by the circadian rhythm. The circadian rhythm is a biological process that regulates the timing of various physiological and behavioral functions, including sleep and wakefulness.

Circadian rhythm sleep disorders can cause a variety of symptoms, including difficulty falling asleep or staying asleep, excessive daytime sleepiness, and changes in the timing of sleep and wakefulness. There are several different types of circadian rhythm sleep disorders, including:

1. Delayed sleep phase disorder: This condition is characterized by a delayed timing of sleep, with individuals typically falling asleep and waking up later than is typical for their age group.

2. Advanced sleep phase disorder: This condition is characterized by an advanced timing of sleep, with individuals typically falling asleep and waking up earlier than is typical for their age group.

3. Shift work disorder: This condition is caused by

working a schedule that is out of sync with the body's natural sleep-wake cycle, such as working overnight shifts.

4. Non-24-hour sleep-wake disorder: This condition is caused by a disruption to the body's circadian rhythm, resulting in a longer-than-normal sleep-wake cycle that is not synchronized with the 24-hour day.

TIPS FOR BETTER SLEEP

The ideal duration for sleep can vary depending on a range of individual factors such as age, lifestyle, and health status. However, in general, most adults require between 7-9 hours of sleep per night to maintain optimal health and well-being.

For children and teenagers, the recommended duration of sleep is generally higher, ranging from 9-12 hours per night for children and 8-10 hours per night for teenagers.

Infants and toddlers require significantly more sleep than older children and adults, as sleep plays a critical role in their physical and cognitive development. Here are some general guidelines for the recommended duration of sleep for infants and toddlers:

1. Newborns (0-3 months): Newborns require a total of 14-17 hours of sleep per day, with individual sleep periods lasting anywhere from 1-4 hours at a time.

2. Infants (4-11 months): Infants require a total of 12-15 hours of sleep per day, typically consisting of several daytime naps and a longer period of nighttime sleep.

3. Toddlers (1-2 years): Toddlers require a total of 11-14 hours of sleep per day, typically consisting of one or two daytime naps and a longer period of nighttime

sleep.

There are a few reasons why it can be harder for adults to fall asleep than children or infants. Here are some of the most common factors that can contribute to difficulty falling asleep in adults:

1. Stress and anxiety: Adults often face more stress and anxiety than children or infants, which can make it difficult to relax and fall asleep. Worries about work, family, or other responsibilities can keep the mind active and make it harder to settle down for sleep.

2. Irregular sleep schedules: Many adults have irregular sleep schedules due to work, social, or other commitments. This can disrupt the body's natural sleep-wake cycle and make it harder to fall asleep and wake up at the desired times.

3. Poor sleep habits: Poor sleep habits such as consuming caffeine or alcohol close to bedtime, engaging in stimulating activities such as using electronic devices, and sleeping in a noisy or uncomfortable environment can all make it harder to fall asleep and stay asleep.

4. Medical conditions: Certain medical conditions such as chronic pain, sleep apnea, and restless leg syndrome can interfere with sleep and make it harder to fall asleep and stay asleep.

5. Aging: As adults age, the natural sleep-wake cycle can become disrupted, making it harder to fall asleep and stay asleep.

Familial natural short sleep is a rare genetic condition that allows affected individuals to function normally with a shorter-than-average amount of sleep. People with this condition are able to function well with as little as 4-6 hours of sleep per night, compared to the recommended 7-9 hours per night for most adults.

The condition is believed to be inherited in an autosomal dominant pattern, meaning that a person only needs to inherit one copy of the gene from either parent to develop the condition. The exact genetic mechanisms underlying familial natural short sleep are not yet fully understood, but researchers have identified several genes that may be involved in regulating sleep duration and quality.

While people with familial natural short sleep may not experience negative consequences from getting less sleep than the average person, it's important to note that most people do require a certain amount of sleep to maintain optimal health and well-being. Chronic sleep deprivation can have negative effects on physical, mental, and emotional health, and can increase the risk of a range of chronic diseases and conditions.

Intentional sleep deprivation refers to the act of voluntarily restricting the amount of sleep an individual gets. This can occur for a variety of reasons, including work, social, or personal obligations, as well as lifestyle factors such as partying or staying up late.

While intentional sleep deprivation may be necessary or desirable in certain circumstances, it's important to note that chronic sleep deprivation can have negative effects on physical, mental, and emotional health, and can increase the risk of a range of chronic diseases and conditions.

Genetics

There have been several studies on sleep duration in **monozygotic (identical) twins** that have compared sleep duration and quality between genetically identical individuals. By comparing sleep patterns in identical twins, researchers can examine the extent to which sleep patterns are influenced by genetic factors versus environmental factors.

One study published in the journal Sleep in 2008 examined the sleep patterns of 1,171 pairs of monozygotic twins and 601 pairs of **dizygotic twins**. The study found that genetic factors accounted for approximately 35% of the variance in total sleep time, suggesting that there is a significant genetic component to sleep duration.

Another study published in the Journal of Sleep Research in 2010 examined the sleep patterns of 32 pairs of monozygotic twins and found that while there was a high degree of similarity in sleep duration and quality between twins, there were also some differences that could not be explained by genetic factors alone.

Besides environmental factors such as lifestyle, work schedules, and other behavioral factors, genetic factors may play a role in sleep patterns and sleep-related behaviors. ABCC9, DEC2, DRD2, and variants near PAX8 and VRK2 are all genes that have been identified as potentially influencing sleep patterns and sleep-related behaviors.

ABCC9 is a gene that has been linked to deep sleep, and may play a role in regulating sleep duration and quality. Variants in this gene have been associated with increased risk of obstructive sleep apnea, a condition characterized by pauses in breathing during sleep.

DEC2 is a gene that has been linked to short sleep duration, and individuals with mutations in this gene have been found to be able to function normally on less sleep than the average person.

DRD2 is a gene that codes for a dopamine receptor, and has been linked to a variety of behaviors and conditions related to reward and motivation, including addiction and sleep disorders such as restless leg syndrome.

Variants near PAX8 and VRK2 have also been linked to sleep patterns and sleep-related behaviors, although the exact mechanisms by which these genes influence sleep are not yet fully understood.

GWAS (genome-wide association study) is a type of genetic analysis that involves scanning the entire genome of an individual to identify genetic variations associated with a particular trait or condition. In the context of sleep, GWAS studies have been conducted to identify genetic factors that may influence sleep patterns and sleep-related behaviors.

In GWAS studies, researchers collect DNA samples from a large number of individuals and use advanced statistical methods to identify genetic variations that are associated with the trait or condition of interest. This approach has been used to identify a number of genetic variations that may be associated with sleep patterns and sleep-related behaviors, including genes related to sleep duration, sleep quality, and susceptibility to sleep disorders.

One notable example of a GWAS study in the field of sleep research is the UK Biobank study, which is a large-scale study that has collected genetic and health data from over 500,000 individuals in the United Kingdom. This study has been used to identify a number of genetic variations associated with sleep patterns and sleep-related behaviors, including genes related to sleep duration, insomnia, and sleep apnea.

Naps

Naps are a brief period of sleep, typically lasting from a few minutes up to an hour or more, that are taken during the day. While napping is often associated with infants and young children, many adults also take naps as a way to supplement their nighttime sleep and increase their overall daily sleep time.

Research has suggested that napping can have a number of potential benefits, including:

1. Increased alertness and productivity: Napping can help combat feelings of fatigue and sleepiness, and can improve cognitive performance and productivity.
2. Improved memory and learning: Napping has been shown to help consolidate memories and improve learning and memory retention.
3. Stress relief: Napping can help reduce feelings of stress and tension, and can promote relaxation and rejuvenation.
4. Improved mood and emotional regulation: Napping can help improve mood and emotional regulation, and can reduce the risk of negative emotional states such as anger and irritability.

Not all individuals may benefit from napping, and that excessive napping can have negative effects on sleep quality and overall health. Additionally, napping at the wrong time or for too long can interfere with nighttime sleep and disrupt the natural sleep-wake cycle.

Sleep inertia refers to the period of grogginess and impaired cognitive performance that may occur immediately upon waking from sleep, particularly after a longer period of sleep or a nap. During sleep, the brain goes through a series of complex physiological and chemical changes that help regulate circadian rhythms and support overall health and well-being. When an individual wakes up, these changes may not immediately reverse, leading to a temporary period of impaired alertness and cognitive performance.

The symptoms of sleep inertia can include feelings of grogginess, confusion, disorientation, impaired motor coordination, and reduced cognitive performance. These symptoms can last for several minutes or longer, depending on individual factors such as the duration and quality of sleep, the time of day, and other environmental and lifestyle factors.

Sleep inertia is particularly common after longer periods of sleep or after taking naps, as the body may be more deeply entrenched in the sleep cycle and have a harder time transitioning to wakefulness. However, sleep inertia can also occur after waking up from shorter periods of sleep or after interrupted sleep.

To minimize the effects of sleep inertia, it can be helpful to follow healthy sleep habits and prioritize regular sleep schedules, as well as to avoid napping for too long or waking up in the middle of a deep sleep cycle. Additionally, engaging in light physical activity or exposure to bright light upon waking can help stimulate the body and promote wakefulness.

Polyphasic sleep is a sleep pattern in which an individual takes several short naps throughout the day, rather than one long period of sleep at night. Proponents of polyphasic sleep argue that it can increase productivity and allow individuals to function on less overall sleep, since the body is given more frequent opportunities to rest and recover.

There are several different polyphasic sleep patterns that individuals may follow, each with its own specific schedule and structure. One common polyphasic sleep pattern is the "Uberman" schedule, in which an individual takes six 20-minute naps throughout the day, for a total of two hours of sleep per day. Another common polyphasic sleep pattern is the "Everyman" schedule, in which an individual takes one longer nap (typically 1.5-2 hours) at night, as well as several shorter naps throughout the day.

While proponents of polyphasic sleep argue that it can increase productivity and reduce the amount of time spent sleeping, there is little scientific evidence to support these claims. Additionally, many individuals may find it difficult to adapt to a polyphasic sleep schedule, as it can be challenging to train the body to sleep in short, intermittent bursts.

Process S

Process S (or the sleep homeostat) is a term used to describe the body's natural mechanism for regulating sleep and wakefulness. The sleep homeostat is responsible for maintaining a balance between the body's need for sleep and its ability to stay awake, and works by accumulating sleep pressure over the course of the day, which is then released during periods of sleep.

Sleep pressure is thought to be related to the accumulation of a molecule called adenosine in the brain, which increases throughout the day and is cleared from the body during sleep. As adenosine levels rise, the body's need for sleep also increases, and the sleep homeostat works to ensure that the body is able to get the rest it needs.

The sleep homeostat is one of several factors that contribute to the regulation of sleep and wakefulness, along with circadian rhythms, environmental factors, and individual lifestyle and behavioral factors.

Sleep deprivation can have a number of negative effects on cognitive and emotional functioning, as well as physical health. Some of the most common effects of sleep deprivation include:

- Slower brain waves in the frontal cortex: Sleep deprivation can lead to a decrease in activity in the prefrontal cortex, the part of the brain responsible for executive functioning, decision-making, and other higher-order cognitive processes.
- Shortened attention span: Sleep deprivation can lead to a decrease in attention and focus, making it harder to stay alert and engaged during the day.
- Higher anxiety: Sleep deprivation can increase feelings of stress and anxiety, making it harder to cope with daily challenges and increasing the risk of mood disorders.
- Impaired memory: Sleep deprivation can interfere with memory consolidation and retrieval, leading to difficulties with learning and retaining information.
- Grouchy mood: Sleep deprivation can cause irritability, moodiness, and other negative emotional states, making it harder to regulate emotions and interact with others.

Adenosine is a naturally occurring chemical that is produced by cells throughout the body, including in the brain. It plays a key role in the regulation of sleep and wakefulness, as well as in other physiological and metabolic processes.

One of the primary functions of adenosine is to signal to the body that it needs rest and sleep. Adenosine levels in the brain increase throughout the day as the body expends energy and resources, creating a sense of fatigue and sleepiness. This process is referred to as the homeostatic sleep drive or sleep pressure, and is one of the primary mechanisms by which the body regulates sleep.

Adenosine exerts its effects on the body by binding to specific receptors in the brain, known as adenosine receptors. When adenosine binds to these receptors, it promotes relaxation and drowsiness, and helps to prepare the body for sleep.

Caffeine, which is found in coffee, tea, and other beverages, works by blocking adenosine receptors in the brain, which can help to increase alertness and wakefulness. However, this effect is only temporary, and caffeine can actually interfere with normal sleep patterns if consumed too close to bedtime.

Natural Ways to Improve Sleep

Here are some tips for better sleep:

1. Stick to a consistent sleep schedule: Go to bed and wake up at the same time every day, even on weekends. This helps regulate your body's internal clock.

2. Create a sleep-conducive environment: Keep your bedroom quiet, cool, and dark. Invest in a comfortable mattress and pillow.

3. Limit caffeine and alcohol: Avoid consuming caffeine

and alcohol close to bedtime, as they can disrupt sleep.

4. Limit screen time before bed: The blue light emitted by electronic devices can interfere with sleep. Try to avoid using electronic devices for at least an hour before bed.

5. Relax before bedtime: Engage in relaxing activities before bed, such as taking a warm bath or practicing relaxation techniques like meditation or deep breathing.

6. Exercise regularly: Regular exercise can help improve sleep quality, but try to avoid vigorous exercise close to bedtime.

7. Don't eat heavy meals before bedtime: Eating heavy or spicy meals close to bedtime can disrupt sleep.

8. Manage stress: Stress and anxiety can interfere with sleep. Try to manage stress with relaxation techniques or seek professional help if necessary.

9. Consider a sleep aid: If you have trouble sleeping, talk to your healthcare professional about sleep aids that may be appropriate for you.

Remember, good sleep is essential to overall health and well-being. Making small changes to your sleep habits can have a big impact on the quality of your sleep and your overall health.

The best time to exercise and the best time to eat may vary depending on individual preferences and daily routines. However, here are some general guidelines that may be helpful.

Morning exercise can be a great way to start the day, as it can help increase energy levels and improve mood throughout the day. However, some people may prefer to exercise in the evening, as it can help relieve stress and anxiety after a long day. The most important thing is to find a time that works for you and your schedule.

It's generally recommended to avoid eating heavy meals close to bedtime, as it can interfere with sleep. However, the timing of meals throughout the day may depend on individual preferences and daily routines. Some people prefer to eat a larger breakfast and a smaller dinner, while others prefer to eat several small meals throughout the day. It's important to listen to your body's hunger and fullness signals and eat in a way that feels satisfying and nourishing.

It is possible to get **too much sleep**. While most people need 7-9 hours of sleep per night to feel rested and refreshed, some people may require more or less sleep. However, consistently sleeping more than 9 hours per night can be a sign of an underlying health condition or lifestyle factor.

Getting too much sleep may lead to a variety of negative effects, including feeling groggy or lethargic, difficulty concentrating, and increased risk of depression and other mood disorders. In some cases, excessive sleep can be a symptom of an underlying health condition, such as sleep apnea, narcolepsy, or depression.

If you find that you consistently need more than 9 hours of sleep per night to feel rested and alert, it may be worth speaking to a healthcare professional to rule out any underlying health conditions or lifestyle factors that may be affecting your sleep.

There are several natural supplements that may be helpful for promoting sleep, including:

1. Melatonin: A hormone produced naturally by the body that helps regulate the sleep-wake cycle.

2. Valerian root: An herb that has been used for centuries as a natural sleep aid. Valerian root may help improve sleep quality and reduce the time it takes to fall asleep.

3. Chamomile: A natural herb that has a calming effect and may help improve sleep quality.

4. Magnesium: A mineral that is essential for a variety of bodily functions, including sleep regulation. Magnesium supplements may be helpful for improving sleep quality and reducing insomnia.

5. Passionflower: An herb that may help reduce anxiety and promote relaxation, making it helpful for improving sleep.

It's important to speak to a healthcare professional before taking any natural supplements, as they may interact with medications or have side effects. Additionally, while natural supplements can be helpful for promoting sleep, they should not be relied on as a substitute for healthy sleep habits and good sleep hygiene.

Melatonin is a hormone produced naturally by the body that helps regulate the sleep-wake cycle. In addition to its role in sleep regulation, melatonin has been studied for its potential effects on the immune system and autoimmune diseases.

Research has suggested that melatonin may have immunomodulatory effects, meaning that it can help regulate the immune system and reduce inflammation. This may be particularly relevant for autoimmune diseases, which occur when the immune system mistakenly attacks healthy tissues in the body.

Some studies have suggested that melatonin may have beneficial effects in individuals with autoimmune diseases, such as rheumatoid arthritis, multiple sclerosis, and lupus. For example, a 2012 study found that melatonin supplementation improved disease activity and symptoms in individuals with rheumatoid arthritis.

However, more research is needed to fully understand the potential benefits of melatonin for autoimmune diseases. It's important to speak to a healthcare professional before taking melatonin or any other supplements, especially if you have an autoimmune disease or are taking medications that may interact with melatonin.

If you are taking immunosuppressant medications, it's important to speak to a healthcare professional before taking melatonin or any other supplements, **as they may interact with your medications and affect their effectiveness**. Your healthcare provider may be able to recommend alternative strategies for improving sleep, or may suggest adjusting your medication regimen to account for any potential interactions.

Most melatonin supplement labels include **warnings** and precautions to be aware of. These warnings may vary depending on the specific product, but some common warnings found on **melatonin labels include**:

1. Not recommended for use by pregnant or breastfeeding women.
2. Not recommended for use by children.
3. May cause drowsiness, so use caution when driving or operating heavy machinery.
4. May interact with certain medications, including blood thinners, blood pressure medications, and

immune suppressants.

5. May cause side effects such as headaches, dizziness, nausea, and irritability in some individuals.

It's important to read and follow the label instructions carefully, and to speak to a healthcare professional before taking melatonin or any other supplements, especially if you have a medical condition, are taking medications, or are pregnant or breastfeeding.

Valerian root supplements usually come with warnings and precautions, and it's important to be aware of these before taking them. Some common warnings that may be found on Valerian root supplement labels include:

1. Not recommended for use by pregnant or breastfeeding women.

2. May cause drowsiness, so use caution when driving or operating heavy machinery.

3. May interact with certain medications, including sedatives, anti-anxiety medications, and antidepressants.

4. May cause side effects such as headaches, dizziness, upset stomach, and dry mouth in some individuals.

5. Not recommended for long-term use, as it may lead to dependence or withdrawal symptoms.

It's important to read and follow the label instructions carefully, and to speak to a healthcare professional before taking Valerian root or any other supplements, especially if you have a medical condition, are taking medications, or are pregnant or breastfeeding.

Here is a brief list of some commonly prescribed sleep medications, their benefits, and warnings:

1. Ambien (zolpidem) - a sedative-hypnotic medication that helps people fall asleep faster and stay asleep longer. Warnings include the potential for drowsiness, impaired coordination, and cognitive impairment, as well as the risk of dependence and withdrawal symptoms.

2. Lunesta (eszopiclone) - a sedative-hypnotic medication that helps people fall asleep faster and stay asleep longer. Warnings include the potential for drowsiness, impaired coordination, and cognitive impairment, as well as the risk of dependence and withdrawal symptoms.

3. Sonata (zaleplon) - a sedative-hypnotic medication that helps people fall asleep faster. Warnings include the potential for drowsiness, impaired coordination, and cognitive impairment, as well as the risk of dependence and withdrawal symptoms.

4. Rozerem (ramelteon) - a medication that works by affecting the body's natural sleep-wake cycle. Warnings include the potential for drowsiness and impaired coordination, as well as the risk of worsening depression symptoms in some individuals.

5. Trazodone - an antidepressant medication that is sometimes prescribed off-label to help people with sleep problems. Warnings include the potential for drowsiness, impaired coordination, and cognitive impairment, as well as the risk of worsening depression symptoms or suicidal thoughts in some individuals.

It's important to follow the label instructions carefully, and to speak to a healthcare professional before taking any prescription medications for sleep, as they may have potential side effects, drug interactions, or other risks to be aware of.

CONCLUSION

In conclusion, sleep is a vital aspect of human health and well-being. It affects every aspect of our lives, including physical health, cognitive function, emotional regulation, and overall quality of life. While sleep problems are common, they can often be addressed through behavioral interventions or medical treatments.

While everyone can suffer from sleep problems, certain groups may be at higher risk, including older adults, individuals with certain medical or mental health conditions, and people who work irregular or long hours. It is important for everyone to prioritize good sleep habits and seek medical evaluation if necessary to ensure that they are getting the restful sleep they need to support their health and well-being.

Sleep disorders are relatively common, affecting millions of people worldwide. According to the American Sleep Association, up to 70 million Americans may have a sleep disorder, while the National Sleep Foundation reports that sleep problems affect up to 45% of the global population.

Insomnia can be treated with a range of approaches, including behavioral interventions, such as cognitive-behavioral therapy for insomnia (CBT-I), and medication. A healthcare professional can help diagnose and treat insomnia, and provide guidance on how to establish healthy sleep habits to promote restful, restorative sleep.

There are many hospitals in the United States that offer specialized sleep clinics and comprehensive treatment programs for people with insomnia. Here are some of the top-ranked hospitals for sleep disorders and insomnia, according to U.S. News & World Report's 2021-2022 rankings:

1. Mayo Clinic - Rochester, Minnesota
2. Stanford Health Care - Stanford, California
3. Cleveland Clinic - Cleveland, Ohio
4. Johns Hopkins Hospital - Baltimore, Maryland
5. Massachusetts General Hospital - Boston, Massachusetts
6. Ronald Reagan UCLA Medical Center - Los Angeles, California
7. NYU Langone Hospitals - New York, New York
8. University of Michigan Hospitals-Michigan Medicine - Ann Arbor, Michigan
9. Brigham and Women's Hospital - Boston, Massachusetts
10. Northwestern Memorial Hospital - Chicago, Illinois

Each of these hospitals has a team of experts in sleep medicine and can offer a range of diagnostic and treatment options for individuals with insomnia and other sleep disorders. It is important to note that insurance coverage and referral requirements may vary, so it is important to check with each hospital before scheduling an appointment.

There are many hospitals around the world that specialize in the diagnosis and treatment of sleep disorders. Here are some of the top-ranked hospitals for sleep medicine outside of the United States, according to Newsweek's 2021 World's Best Hospitals list:

1. Charité - Universitätsmedizin Berlin (Germany)
2. Assistance Publique – Hôpitaux de Paris (France)
3. Universitätsklinikum Zürich (Switzerland)
4. University of Tokyo Hospital (Japan)
5. Hospital Clínic Barcelona (Spain)
6. Singapore General Hospital (Singapore)
7. King's College Hospital (United Kingdom)
8. Toronto General Hospital (Canada)
9. St. Vincent's Hospital Sydney (Australia)
10. San Raffaele Hospital (Italy)

These hospitals have specialized sleep centers that provide comprehensive diagnosis and treatment for sleep disorders, including insomnia, sleep apnea, and narcolepsy. Each hospital may have different protocols, insurance requirements, and referral procedures, so it is important to research and contact each hospital directly for more information.

ACKNOWLEDGEMENT

Book cover created by Dan Wilson: Image is public domain (Resting Girl by Alexei Harlamov, 1925)

Book sources are listed throughout the book. Here are the ones I used the most:

1. "Why We Sleep: Unlocking the Power of Sleep and Dreams" by Matthew Walker (2017, Scribner) - This book explores the science behind sleep, including the different stages of sleep, the benefits of sleep, and the consequences of sleep deprivation.

2. "The Sleep Solution: Why Your Sleep is Broken and How to Fix It" by W. Chris Winter (2017, Berkley) - This book offers practical tips and advice for improving sleep, including strategies for falling asleep, staying asleep, and waking up feeling refreshed.

3. "Say Good Night to Insomnia: The Six-Week, Drug-Free Program Developed At Harvard Medical School" by Gregg D. Jacobs (2009, Holt Paperbacks) - This book provides a step-by-step program for overcoming insomnia without medication, including techniques for relaxation, cognitive therapy, and lifestyle changes.

4. "Sleep Smarter: 21 Essential Strategies to Sleep Your Way to A Better Body, Better Health, and Bigger Success" by Shawn Stevenson (2016, Rodale Books) - This book provides practical strategies for optimizing sleep, including tips for improving

sleep quality, creating a sleep-conducive environment, and developing a consistent sleep routine.

5. "The Power of When: Discover Your Chronotype--and the Best Time to Eat Lunch, Ask for a Raise, Have Sex, Write a Novel, Take Your Meds, and More" by Michael Breus (2016, Little, Brown and Company) - This book explores the impact of chronotype on sleep and other aspects of life, and offers personalized strategies for optimizing sleep and productivity based on individual sleep patterns.

Study sources:

1. "Sleep and the COVID-19 pandemic" by Altevogt et al. (2021), published in Sleep Health. This study explores the impact of the COVID-19 pandemic on sleep, including changes in sleep patterns, sleep quality, and sleep disorders.

2. "Sleep disturbance and risk of cognitive decline in older adults" by Harrison et al. (2021), published in Sleep Medicine Reviews. This study reviews the evidence linking sleep disturbances to cognitive decline in older adults, and discusses potential mechanisms underlying this association.

3. "Sleep and mental health in college students: a review of empirical research" by Gress-Smith et al. (2020), published in Sleep Health. This study reviews the literature on the relationship between sleep and mental health in college students, including the prevalence of sleep disorders and the impact of poor sleep on mental health outcomes.

4. "Sleep duration and risk of type 2 diabetes: a meta-analysis of prospective studies" by Cai et al. (2021), published in Sleep Medicine. This study reviews the existing evidence on the association between sleep duration and risk of type

2 diabetes, and provides a quantitative synthesis of the findings.

5. "The impact of sleep on pain: a review and synthesis of recent literature" by Goodin et al. (2020), published in Current Psychiatry Reports. This study reviews the recent literature on the bidirectional relationship between sleep and pain, and discusses the potential mechanisms underlying this association.

www.ingramcontent.com/pod-product-compliance
Lightning Source LLC
Chambersburg PA
CBHW061555250726
48657CB00021B/1770